Helen Rehr, DSW
Gary Rosenberg, PhD

The Social Work–Medicine Relationship
100 Years at Mount Sinai

More pre-publication
REVIEWS, COMMENTARIES, EVALUATIONS . . .

"In this engaging book that commemorates the anniversary of 100 years of groundbreaking and important work at the Social Work Department of Mount Sinai, Rehr and Rosenberg draw attention to the innumerable contributions of women (both volunteers and professionals), the advantage of interdisciplinary professional partnerships, and the significance and impact of innovative and creative programs grounded in hands-on clinical experience and evidence-based practice research. Many 'lessons learned' put forth in this instructive book can be helpful to community-based health care systems as they take steps to address the call for far greater accountability while assisting more diverse and vulnerable groups of people requiring support and services with inadequate and decreasing extant resources and opportunities."

Andrew W. Safyer, PhD
Dean and Professor
Adelphi University
School of Social Work

"The authors, both legendary trailblazers in health care social work, provide a comprehensive overview (colored by their personal and professional experiences in one academic medical center) of the contemporary and historical connection between medicine and social work. Rehr and Rosenberg have made a unique contribution to social work scholarship through their lively and fascinating narrative of this history. The book is particularly valuable in tracing, for the first time, the socialization of an academic medical center by a cadre of women activists who initiated and developed the department of social work. Readers, facing the challenges of social work practice in the twenty-first century, will be reinvigorated and inspired by the comprehensive social-health care philosophies of both past and present leaders in health care social work presented in this volume."

Goldie Kadushin, PhD
Associate Professor
Helen Bader School of Social Work
University of Wisconsin-Milwaukee

"Written by two legendary social work leaders in health, this book gives us an inside look at the development and work of a major center of social work leadership in hospital and community settings. Of greater significance is the comprehensive look at the changing context in America, the evolving role of social work in health, the resounding theme of the need to move from the medical model to the social-health care model. Weaving in the key partnership with exceptional physician leaders, the role of the Auxiliary, the role of women and the move to specialization, these authors have painted a valuable picture of the past. This study in history demonstrates the need for great leaders, for great practitioners, and for the continuous evolution of the vision and the long-term nature of the work of advancing a new paradigm for our health system. It is a valuable work, which sets our work in a framework of change and courageous innovation that is especially helpful in these challenging times."

W. June Simmons, LCSW
President and CEO
Partners in Care Foundation

More pre-publication
REVIEWS, COMMENTARIES, EVALUATIONS . . .

"This book represents a major contribution to literature in the health care field. *The Social Work–Medicine Relationship: 100 Years at Mount Sinai* is much more than a study of the history of medical social work in a major hospital in a large urban area. This book comprehensively explores the history, policy, practice, and research issues in health care, medical social work, and community medicine. This book has something for everyone: administrators, policymakers, educators, researchers, and program developers. This book also is of special benefit to beginning social work practitioners who are struggling with how to understand their role in a complex medical system. It should be on the shelf of every health care provider because of its focus on interdisciplinary work. It should be on the shelf of every social worker, because social workers in all fields of practice see clients with health or health-related issues.

The Social Work–Medicine Relationship: 100 Years at Mount Sinai is particularly valuable at a time when the health care field in general and medical social work in particular is under siege with escalating costs and increasing demands with more older and immigrant patients. This book is not only timely, but future oriented in its description of international programs as we move more to a focus on global issues. At a time when many social work programs in hospitals have either been eliminated or significantly diminished, one can ask why certain programs, such as social work at Mount Sinai, have not only survived but thrived. The secret that the authors so aptly describe is 'developing innovative programs in partnership with health care colleagues and the community.' This approach is apparent throughout the book in the discussion of what visionary leaders have done to promote the practice of social work in health care. In recent years social work in health care has had to revamp its focus from inpatient care to ambulatory and community care. Rather than decry the change and portray it as diminishing the quality of social work, this book describes how social workers among all health care providers are experts in psychosocial and community factors that impact on clients and can make ample use of their specialized knowledge and skills to promote the health and well-being of clients.'

Elaine Congress, DSW
Associate Dean and Professor
Fordham University
Graduate School of Social Service

The Haworth Press
New York • London • Oxford

NOTES FOR PROFESSIONAL LIBRARIANS AND LIBRARY USERS

This is an original book title published by The Haworth Press, Inc. Unless otherwise noted in specific chapters with attribution, materials in this book have not been previously published elsewhere in any format or language.

CONSERVATION AND PRESERVATION NOTES

All books published by The Haworth Press, Inc., and its imprints are printed on certified pH neutral, acid-free book grade paper. This paper meets the minimum requirements of American National Standard for Information Sciences-Permanence of Paper for Printed Material, ANSI Z39.48-1984.

The Social Work–Medicine Relationship
100 Years at Mount Sinai

HAWORTH Social Work in Health Care
Gary Rosenberg and Andrew Weissman
Editors

A Guide to Creative Group Programming in the Psychiatric Day Hospital by Lois E. Passi

Social Work in Geriatric Home Health Care: The Blending of Traditional Practice with Cooperative Strategies by Lucille Rosengarten

Health Care and Empowerment Practice in the Black Community: Knowledge, Skills, and Collectivism by Sadye L. Logan and Edith M. Freeman

Clinical Case Management for People with Mental Illness: A Vulnerability-Stress Model by Daniel Fu Keung Wong

The Social Work–Medicine Relationship: 100 Years at Mount Sinai by Helen Rehr and Gary Rosenberg

The Social Work–Medicine Relationship
100 Years at Mount Sinai

Helen Rehr, DSW
Gary Rosenberg, PhD

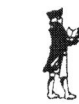

The Haworth Press
New York • London • Oxford

For more information on this book or to order, visit
http://www.haworthpress.com/store/product.asp?sku=5717

or call 1-800-HAWORTH (800-429-6784) in the United States and Canada
or (607) 722-5857 outside the United States and Canada

or contact orders@HaworthPress.com

© 2006 by The Haworth Press, Inc. All rights reserved. No part of this work may be reproduced or utilized in any form or by any means, electronic or mechanical, including photocopying, microfilm, and recording, or by any information storage and retrieval system, without permission in writing from the publisher. Printed in the United States of America.

The Haworth Press, Inc., 10 Alice Street, Binghamton, NY 13904-1580.

PUBLISHER'S NOTES
The development, preparation, and publication of this work has been undertaken with great care. However, the Publisher, employees, editors, and agents of The Haworth Press are not responsible for any errors contained herein or for consequences that may ensue from use of materials or information contained in this work. The Haworth Press is committed to the dissemination of ideas and information according to the highest standards of intellectual freedom and the free exchange of ideas. Statements made and opinions expressed in this publication do not necessarily reflect the views of the Publisher, Directors, management, or staff of The Haworth Press, Inc., or an endorsement by them.

Unless otherwise specified, quoted materials that appear in this book were obtained from confidential sources whose identities were protected as a condition of their participation in the research study.

Cover design by Kerry E. Mack.

Library of Congress Cataloging-in-Publication Data

Rehr, Helen.
  The social work–medicine relationship : 100 years at Mount Sinai / Helen Rehr, Gary Rosenberg.
     p. ; cm.
  Includes bibliographical references and index.
  ISBN-13: 978-0-7890-3076-4 (hard : alk. paper)
  ISBN-10: 0-7890-3076-4 (hard : alk. paper)
  ISBN-13: 978-0-7890-3077-1 (soft : alk. paper)
  ISBN-10: 0-7890-3077-2 (soft : alk. paper)
    1. Mount Sinai Hospital (New York, N.Y.). Dept. of Social Work Services—History. 2. Medical social work—New York (State)—New York—History.   I. Rosenberg, Gary. II. Title.
  [DNLM: 1. Mount Sinai Hospital (New York, N.Y.). Dept. of Social Work Services. 2. Community Health Services—history. 3. Social Work Department, Hospital—history.   WX 28 AN7 M928R 2006]

HV688.U6N53 2006
362.12'09747'1—dc22

2005017697

CONTENTS

Foreword ix
    Kenneth L. Davis

**Chapter 1. Introduction: Social Work Services
in Health Care: The Challenges** 1

Chapter 2. Early Medicine and the Social Services 7

**Chapter 3. American Medicine and the Emergence
of the Social Work Profession** 17

    Introduction 17
    Social Work Emerges 20
    Social Work Connects to Medicine 20

**Chapter 4. Mount Sinai Medicine and the Women
Who Socialized the Institution** 33

    The Mount Sinai Auxiliary Board 37
    Summary 42

**Chapter 5. Social Work Activist-Leaders: The Making
of a Social Work Department** 47

    Background 48

Chapter 6. Social Work's Past Shapes the Present 63

    Introduction 63
    An Experiment in Staff Education Conducted at the Social
    Service Department of The Mount Sinai Hospital:
    A 1932 Perspective 64
        Fanny L. Mendelsohn
    A Comprehensive Approach to Social Service
    in a Health Agency: A 1955 Perspective 69
        Doris Siegel

Chapter 7. Social Work Research in Health Care: Studies That Affect Practice — 85

Premise — 86
Background — 87
Social Work Studies Itself — 90
An Aspiring Researcher Begins at Mount Sinai — 97
Barbara Berkman
Thirty-Five Years of Social Work at Elmhurst Hospital — 99
Lawrence Cuzzi
From Evaluation Methodologist to Clinical Data-Miner: Finding Treasure Through Practice-Based Research — 101
Irwin Epstein
Going Across Town and Out into the World — 107
Gary Holden
Conclusion — 111

Chapter 8. Community Medicine and the Social Work Connection — 113

Background — 114
The Division of Social Work — 117
Social Work Role in Medical Education — 118
Schools of Social Work — 120
Community Practice — 121
Research — 123
Conclusion — 124

Chapter 9. The Globalization of Social Work Services in Social-Health Care — 127

An International Exchange Among Social Work Leaders — 127
The Enhanced Leadership Program — 130
The Needs of Developing Countries — 138
The Needs of Western Social Workers — 140
Other Enhancement of Leadership Programs — 141

Chapter 10. Medicine and Social Work: The Social-Health Challenge — 143

The Economics of Health Care Delivery — 144
The New Millennium — 147

Social Work and Social Policy	150
Tomorrow's Social Work	155
Conclusions	160

Appendix I. Directors, Department of Social Work Service — 165

Appendix II. Edith J. Baerwald Professors of Community Medicine (Social Work) and Chairpersons, Division of Social Work and Behavioral Sciences — 167

Appendix III. Chairpersons, Auxiliary Board — 169

Appendix IV. Social Work Events — 171

Appendix V. Auxiliary Board Projects, 1969 to 2004 — 177

Appendix VI. Women As Volunteers — 181
   Introduction — 181
   A Personal History of an Auxiliary Board Member — 182
      Hortense Hirsch

References — 191

Index — 201

ABOUT THE AUTHORS

Helen Rehr, DSW, has had a career of over fifty years at The Mount Sinai Medical Center, holding a range of practice, research, teaching, and administrative positions. Dr. Rehr was the Director of the Department of Social Work and the Director of the Division of Social Work (Department of Community and Preventive Medicine) at the Mount Sinai School of Medicine. Dr. Rehr is an Adjunct Clinical Professor at Hunter College School of Social Work and the Brookdale Center on Aging. She has held visiting professorships in Israel and Australia. Dr. Rehr is the author, co-author, and editor of over 100 published studies, reports, monographs, articles, chapters, and books, and continues her editorial board membership with Social Work in Health Care, which has created a prestigious annual award in her name. Dr. Rehr was the recipient of the Ida M. Cannon Award, the highest award of the Society of Hospital Social Work Directors of the American Hospital Association.

Gary Rosenberg, PhD, is the Edith J. Baerwald Professor of Community and Preventive Medicine at the Mount Sinai School of Medicine. He is the past President of the Society for Social Work Administrators in Health Care. Dr. Rosenberg has been elected to the Hunter College Hall of Fame and has received the Distinguished Alumni Award from Adelphi University and the Founders Day Award from New York University. In addition, he is a Fellow in the Brookdale Center on Aging, a Fellow in the New York Academy of Medicine, and a recipient of the Ida M. Cannon Award of the Society for Hospital Social Work Directors of the American Hospital Association.

Foreword

As the administrative leader of The Mount Sinai Medical Center, I have both the privilege and challenge of following in the footsteps of Dr. S. S. Goldwater, the first professional medical administrator in the United States. It was under Dr. Goldwater's leadership that The Mount Sinai Hospital formed the Social Service Department—the third in the nation.

Dr. Goldwater wrote, "The most important person in the hospital is not the governor, the contributor, the doctor, the nurse, the superintendent, or the secretary; the most important person in the hospital, beyond all question, is the patient." This simple yet poignant philosophy led him in 1906 to approve the founding of the Social Service Department because he was convinced that it would contribute directly to better care of patients.*

As much of a visionary as Dr. Goldwater was, it is hard to imagine that he could have predicted just how dramatic the benefit to patients would be. In the century since he made this momentous decision, health care in the United States has undergone dramatic change.

The dynamics of today's physician-patient relationship bare little resemblance to such interactions at the dawn of the last century. In the early 1900s, most physicians lived and worked in the same community as their patients. Home visits were routine. The doctor got to know patients within many and varied contexts. In today's more mobile world, in which medical science has become far more complex, the relationship between doctor and patient is condensed into limited time within an office or hospital.

Parallel to the narrowing of the physician-patient relationship, the social and economic factors that impact a patient's care have become

---

*From *The First Hundred Years of The Mount Sinai Hospital of New York 1852-1952* by Joseph Hirsch and Beka Doherty. Published by Random House, New York.

far more complex. Disparities in insurance coverage, financial resources, living conditions, family support systems, and countless other areas directly impact patient care. Finding one's way through the mountains of red tape and paperwork needed to find and receive critical services has become nearly impossible for an individual without special training.

Although physicians today have arsenals of technology and drugs to which to turn for treating almost every disease, these remain far from sufficient to treat the patient, who is, after all, far more than his or her disease. The physician and the social worker must as a team consider all the factors that impact a patient's health and devise the best course of treatment based on the individual's needs.

Within my own medical specialty of psychiatry, I have had ample opportunity to learn firsthand the necessity and benefits of physicians and social workers partnering to care for patients. We are fortunate today to have far greater understanding of the complex workings of the human brain than any previous generation. As a result, many conditions previously thought hopeless are manageable. However, no manner of drug or psychotherapy can assist a patient whose disease has already stripped him or her of basic necessities such as access to food and shelter. First and foremost, such patients must receive the assistance a social worker can provide; then, and only then, medical interventions can help.

Such a dramatic scenario is but one small example of the myriad ways in which doctors and social workers need each other in order to achieve their common goal of helping the patient.

Beyond the individual patient, communities and, indeed, society as a whole also must be viewed simultaneously through the lenses of the social worker and the physician if we hope to prevent disease and improve health. Physicians working in isolation may develop masterful prevention strategies; however, without an understanding of the social fabric in which these strategies must be implemented, they are but plans on worthless paper with little hope of success.

From its roots doing outreach to care for our poorest patients, the role of social work at Mount Sinai has expanded exponentially. Social work programs and research conducted at Mount Sinai not only impact our patients, they impact our community, our state, our nation, and our world.

As you read through this book and learn of the challenges encountered and the contributions made by social work professionals over the last century, I'm sure you will realize, as I do, that we all owe an enormous debt of gratitude to the men and women who built this magnificent partnership between medicine and social work.

Kenneth L. Davis, MD
President & CEO,
Mount Sinai Medical Center;
Dean,
Mount Sinai School of Medicine

Chapter 1

Introduction: Social Work Services in Health Care: The Challenges

Social work, the profession, is being pulled in many directions. As social work developed, finding new and essential roles and functions in multiple fields, the profession took on many modes. Over time the clinical and social policy arenas separated (as did medicine from public health), and the academics and the practitioners did not find unity. As each division tended to serve itself, the result was professional separation rather than togetherness. In addition, the incursion of behaviorists and nurses into counseling roles, interprofessional turf conflicts, deprofessionalization, and the commercialization of health care services have led to an uncertainty in social work roles and direction. But the major impacts come from the unpredictability of fiscal support for the social services, from the still uncertain status of social work in health settings, and from a continuing lack of social work visibility and understanding of its benefits by the public, administrators, payers, and regulators.

The current economic crisis is affecting the employment market, the social welfare system, health care services, and education for professional practice as a result of severe cutbacks in support by government and private insurers for service delivery. In addition, government support of public social-health policy has been eroding in the last decade. The health care insurance companies have either not incorporated social service benefit into their policies or have limited social services benefits. Another drawback is that social work has not transmitted an adequate message of its benefits and its availability to those in need in health care and to those who are vulnerable in coping with illness and/or disorders, irrespective of economic status.

Those in low-income groups and those in poverty are generally perceived by the public based on the country's economic status. When the country is affluent, the populace tends to be more generous in offering help to those in need. When the country is fiscally unstable, the populace believes the poor should help themselves. It appears that economics governs the availability of accessible medical care as well as health care social services. What is essential is a social-health policy regarding the "right to health care" and affordable comprehensive care. Although social work is responsible for the majority of mental health counseling services to those with biopsychosocial problems, the profession as organized in social or health agencies has not made its benefits sufficiently known to cause a public demand for social work services and for the support for serving those with social-health needs. Conservative beliefs about the moral causes of poverty affect public policies and lead to increasing numbers of persons in the United States who are uninsured or underinsured. Emphasis is still placed on illness, and very little attention is given to support primary prevention and health promotion throughout the life cycle.

In addition, most people agree that the current American health care delivery system is bleeding. The past two decades of cost containment, competition, and deregulation have barely controlled the hemorrhaging of a system that may be the world's most sophisticated yet still costs too much and does not serve all who need care. American health care is a paradox of excess and deprivation. Excess occurs when people with comprehensive health insurance receive unnecessary and inappropriate health services. Deprivation occurs when those who are poor and those without insurance or with inadequate insurance are denied care. After the debacle of a prospective universal health care policy in the 1990s, politicians may again be interested in responding to the public's concern about the rising cost of medical care and its quality.

We have come from a century in which vast changes have occurred. From its beginnings of a nonmedical care system in America and the country's early social tumult, we have seen the development of a medical care system, a public health system, and a social welfare system amid tumultuous waves of economic growth and temporary declines. The 1900s have also spawned the development of American social work as a profession. In the latter half of the twentieth century, those whose social work life span is included in this period have seen societal needs and expectations impacting the health care system and its practitioners. The development of new organizational arrangements, technology, and enhanced medical and surgical practices have also changed the delivery of care. Yet, with all the advancements, more in the twentieth century than in all prior centuries combined, neither government nor science has resolved the ongoing problems relevant to disease, hunger, poverty, and those surfacing today such as AIDS, abuse, and violence and their impact on individual and family life.

Although there have been major advances and an improved public health system as we have entered the new century, the current government has moved to diminish its support of the means to the "right to health care" of its citizens. Inequality in availability, affordability, and access to care remains, as it affects different groups: those with low income, minorities, noncitizens, and the homeless. In shifting the political direction from social-health care as a public social utility to commercialized enterprises, the balance of power and planning has moved to a corporate presence exercising medical determination. The shift has reduced the availability of professional diagnosis and treatment and social-health care for many and has placed the burden of responsibility for support and care on the individual person and his or her social network with less help and professional assistance.

While many of the social-health problems of the past century remain today, many gains have affected medical care that need to be recognized and that affect social work in health care. Some of these gains include the following:

- a provision of patient's rights in his or her medical care;
- informed consent as an essential component of care;
- the scientific and technological advances that have dealt with diseases and other treatments;
- the enactment of multiple health insurance programs, e.g., Medicare, Medicaid;
- the development of rehabilitation medicine;
- a biopsychosocial approach to dealing with illness and disorders;
- a social-health model of care versus a medical model;
- a lay public participation in medical institutional programs, initiated by the Model Cities Act;

- peer review and accountability of quality care;
- legalization of abortion, as a woman's right;
- the growth of consumers', women's, and the civil rights movements;
- end-of-life decision making as an individual determination;
- self-help groups to assist individuals with specific diseases;
- the development of national organizations and foundations to deal with disease/disorder entities; and
- the use of the Internet as a health-informative tool, which reduces professional consultations.

Health care has shifted from an essentially voluntary, insurance, employer-employee benefit and government-supported system to a deregulated, competitive commercialized enterprise. Today's managed care and commercial insurers with their capped benefits and prescribed cost reimbursements tend to be cost control and profit oriented organizations. Prevention and health maintenance coverage is rarely included in their policies. Public health services remain underfunded and lacking in direction. Health care is focused on illness treatment and limited on prevention. There is not enough emphasis on the populations at risk and the health needs within given communities.

It is today's health care, its availability, affordability, and quality that remain the public's concern. The beginning of the new century introduces a health care delivery system in crisis. It is difficult to predict the future in meeting the social and health care services needed and in making available an affordable and accessible care system for all Americans. The key concerns are what care will be available, "who" will provide "what," and "how" will care be paid. We enter the twenty-first century recognizing the past and knowing much remains to be done to create a comprehensive social-health care system with affordable service coverage. It will require a multiprofessional force supported by quality education of the different disciplines.

Is there meaning today in writing a history of medicine and the social work connection? If one looks at the history of medicine, one sees the different means of supporting the sick in early times by tribes, societies, and the church as well as some of the horrific dealings such as eliminating the sick. However, whatever emerged over time, charitable help was in evidence from the beginning of recorded history.

Many years ago, one of the authors sat in a class given by Dr. Albert Lyons on the history of medicine. She then read the Lyons and Petrucelli book *Medicine: An Illustrated History* and looked for a comparable illustrated history of the social services (or their equivalent) and could not find any similar approach to social work's past. In the 1940s, having done a history of medical education and social work's role for class, that exercise whetted her curiosity about social work's past. After all these years, we started to look back.

What the authors have attempted is an overview of medicine past and present and how social work and committed women have connected to medical care, its institutions, and the health needs of populations at risk. It reflects on the authors' views, each looking back after fifty and thirty years in the social services in one medical center. Such looking back and ahead is colored by personal, professional experiences in an organization that has undergone multiple leaderships and changes over fifty years—the latter half of the twentieth century and into the beginning of the twenty-first century. In touching on the past, the authors have generalized to given historical periods, reflecting on the relationship of the social services to medicine. In a way social and environmental support for the sick has been available from the beginning of the practice to aid the sick. (See Kerson, 1981, for the relationship of societal work and social events.)

Much has happened in the field of medicine. It has advanced with more medical innovations during the twentieth century than in all past centuries combined. Yet medicine remains on the cusp with more to conquer. Although many diseases and disorders may be tempered by research, innovation, and public health measures, much of what exists today in the way of disease and disorder is expected to be at least into the next twenty-five years. The way people use professional medical care is changing. Although more partnership occurs between patient and physician, there is more use of technology via the Internet. A mountain of information is available on the Internet—freely available. The concern remains as to how to make its use sound and safe as long as interpretation and consultation services are lacking or not utilized.

The authors have decided to introduce the development of social work services and medicine in one academic medical center in reflecting on the gains and the losses. In so doing they hope to portray the social work relationship to medicine over a fifty-year period in an attempt to demonstrate the accomplishments gained in serving its patients and its community. Quality leadership, visionary laywomen, administrative groups, and fiscal responsibility led to innovations in comprehensive care, which shaped a model of social-health care replacing the traditional medical model of service. Many advances served to fulfill the institution's missions. One example is the relationship of social work and medicine.

In the past ten years societal changes—social, medical, political, demographic, and economic—have been many. They have affected the patterns of medical care in the institution where these authors served in practice, administrative, educational, and research roles. The fiscal impact on health care has had a negative effect on the quality, the availability, and the access of care for all prospective clientele. Institutions across the country have been forced to cut back on their programs. The public is aware of the problems in the delivery of quality health care and has registered its concern about the medical care available to it.

The changes have undoubtedly influenced our perceptions of the past and of today's events and led to speculations on tomorrow's American social-health care system.

Will there be a universal comprehensive social-health care policy with entitlements for all Americans? Will social work be active in providing services and in advocating for a social-health policy for those in need?

Chapter 2

Early Medicine and the Social Services

Social work is in a sense "ancient history." Medical history offers social work in health care a perspective on what people undertook in caring for those with social-health needs. Sufficient evidence indicates that disease existed in prehistoric times. Archaeological finds of human remains suggest evidence of fractures, inflammation, and other physical irregularities. The question that has been posed by anthropologists is "was there a cult of healing" to deal with these recognized anomalies. As humans moved from "food gathering" to "food producing," there appears to be indication of the development of medicinal herbs. It is known that spiritual ritual—culturally based—was a significant factor toward treating ailments. However, much of caring in early times appeared to be self-directed.

As primitive cultures have been studied, the supernatural was believed to affect all things. Humans separated their daily, ordinary practices and conditions from those that appeared to be different and unusual, as induced by "evil" forces. These latter required special assistance from a medicine man, a shaman, or a witch doctor. The individual afflicted and the healer perceived a supernatural causation. They were together in being "psychologically" invested by a magic to deal with the trauma (Lyons and Petrucelli, 1978, p. 3). Different cultures had different perceptions for the course of illness, sickness, disability, and mental illness, ranging from good to bad spirits. Some acted by shunning the afflicted and others by killing off the disabled or the old.

There were those who were "healers" who ministered to the sick. Healers could have multiple functions such as protecting the harvest or inducing a special event, or they could be specialized dealers for given symptoms and ailments that affected a body part. Illness was seen as caused by gods, spirits, and magic affecting the individual who it was believed brought the affliction on himself because of misdeeds. A history of the "happening" related to the problem was the instrument used by the healer in order to mitigate the affliction. The healer's armamentarium could include medicinal plants, hallucinatory drugs, salves for infections, and even a form of surgery to deal with wounds or injured bones. Over time, trial and error of treatments led to further use of mineral substances and even to the use of "heat" for given conditions. What was most significant was the recognition by those entrusted with the healing function that a "psychological" benefit was induced in the sick by the very act of doing something. Magic was the cure for supernatural causes. Observation by healers led them to recognize that some conditions did not strike twice and to understand that certain conditions self-healed. As observations increased and were shared, it was noted that given conditions were frequent occurrences. Some cultures introduced common means to deal with given conditions such as public health measures, e.g., the introduction of latrines and the drainage of wastes.

As early as 1700 BC in ancient civilization, there is a record of the regulation of the practice of medicine (Lyons and Petrucelli, 1978, p. 59). Illness was still perceived as supernaturally imposed, but it was now attributable to sin or misdeeds. Prayers and sacrifices were the common religious means to assuage the gods in seeking cures. Medicines were already in use and noted for given conditions. The healers were now classified by function and/or beliefs. There were those who "diagnosed" (symptoms only) and those who "treated"; exorcists were healer-types who used charms, divination, drugs, and even surgery (Lyons and Petrucelli, 1978, p. 67). Healers were educated in priestly temples. Symptoms had begun to be classified, not as diseases but based on their location, e.g., chest, abdomen. By this time, there was a separation of care for the rich undertaken by these priestly healers and for the poor by the equivalent of barbers.

The biblical Hebrews held the belief that disease was "divine punishment" for a committed sin. The Hebrews differed from other sects in that their beliefs were monotheistic rather than polytheistic or spiritual. The Bible and the Talmud offer a rich medical lore influenced by the Greek philosophers who had some knowledge of anatomy and physiology and who used diet, drugs, massage (Lyons and Petrucelli, 1978, p. 72), surgery, and bloodletting. The mores required one individual to serve another in times of need. Organized religion fostered this concept in the broad application of brotherhood and "serve thy neighbor." The Hebrews added a form of public health to their doctrines, which included dietary practices and cleanliness. Although immersion was considered a means of purification from sin, it was also a factor in cleanliness. The early Christians adopted baptism by rites of immersion (from Hebrew law) as early as the first century (Cahill, 1999, p. 122). Other early documentation included "teaching" materials, a sort of regulation of medical to-dos.

It is not known when hospitals as such were designed. Some evidence suggests that types of dispensaries with specific functions, such as for maternity care in ancient India, were in place as early as the third century BC (Lyons and Petrucelli, 1978, p. 119). In ancient China evidence supports that prevention was a major practice. Such factors as temperance, simplicity in lifestyle, and sexual mores were philosophically prescribed. Diagnosis was based on both physiological examination and explicit learning about the patient from the patient. Treatment of illnesses included medicines, acupuncture, and exercise, but could also include foot binding, castration, and a variety of divinely prescribed modalities.

As hospitals were created, they were more like hospices for the sick poor, staffed by priest-physicians. Upper-class individuals when ill were also treated by priest-physicians, but essentially at home. In China, there was a sort of "accountability" system wherein doctors had to report both successes and failures (Lyons and Petrucelli, 1978, p. 141). A ranking as to quality levels was developed and publicly known by the elite. Chinese medicine was well developed early, including schools for medical education. The education for medical practice moved to the East as early as the seventh and eighth centuries. Personal examinations were required in order to qualify to be a physician as early as the seventh century AD (Lyons and Petrucelli, 1978, p. 141).

In Greece, while the gods were thought to induce illness, there was evidence of knowledge of anatomy and physiology competing with superstition. The Greeks introduced the tenet that a "life force" emanated from inside the body and also that the "psyche" was "the soul or individual personality" (Lyons and Petrucelli, 1978, p. 154). The Greeks created "temples" or "spas" associated with dealing with illness and also to support health maintenance. Programs included diet, exercise, divination, medication, immersions, and magic. The key catalyst, however, was "faith" as the curing medium. "Health" spas live on today with the same objective.

While information for caring for sickness was passed on orally by itinerant craftsmen, schools had begun to develop in the Mediterranean areas. Science-philosophers were in place developing treatises, attitudes, and disease categories and related treatments. Much of the developments stemmed from the initial concepts of medicine developed by Hippocrates (b. 470 BC), who had already produced treatises dealing with a conceptualization of general beliefs including anatomy, physiology, diagnosis, and prognosis. Mental illness was recognized in the context of depression, anxiety, and epilepsy, and even dreams were noted as an ailment. A code of behavior and ethics for practitioners had been promulgated calling for holding confidences of patients and being committed against their harm and injustice. The Hippocratic method included observation, a study of the patient (not the disease), assessment, and attempts to assist nature while drawing on the body's natural forces (Lyons and Petrucelli, 1978, pp. 216-217) and to do "no harm." Galen (129-200 AD), a Greek physician-scientist who wrote extensively based on his practice and whose works carried into the Middle Ages, was endorsed by both Christians and Muslims. The code and methods (although limited then) as doctrine led to the concept of the whole person in his or her environment.

Early Roman medicine was comparable to the early Greek medicine. However, the Romans were contributing to medical knowledge well into the first and second centuries AD. They were also public health conscious in constructing aqueducts for their water system. The Romans, a warlike people, created hostels for the care of the wounded military on fields of battle.

Before Christ, the poor sick were seen as unworthy in most primitive cultures; theirs was a self-care or care via a tribal ritual. Christianity, sometime in the fourth century, interprets a Christlike mission of healing. Facilities are begun to be established to care for the sick and oppressed, i.e., the poor, elderly, foundlings, orphans, and the downfallen (Lyons and Petrucelli, 1978, p. 272). A "hospital" is founded for these vulnerable groups about 330 AD. In 369 AD the first Christian public hospitals for care of plague victims is founded in Europe and in Bethlehem. Christian hospices devoted to long-term care of the poor and the downtrodden were sustained by the "good" women of noble birth whose function was essentially that of caretaking (Lyons and Petrucelli, 1978, p. 272). After Rome fell to the Goths in 476 AD, the Dark Ages ensued when much of caretaking fell by the wayside, leaving individuals to care for themselves.

The Arabic world, influenced by the Greeks, Romans, and the Jews, contributed much to medicine. Arabs were great collectors of data, adding to the sciences and to pharmacopoeia. Islam encouraged scholars from the non-Muslim world—accepting Jewish and Greek physicians without prejudice. The most famous Jewish physician in Arabic medicine was Maemonides (1135-1204 AD), who practiced in Morocco, Palestine, and Cairo. Islam is credited with the development of the modern hospital system. The best were in Baghdad, Damascus, and Cairo. The latter included teaching centers, libraries, separate wards for different diseases, and convalescent sections. After-care was a major concern as evidenced on discharge, when patients received five gold pieces to support themselves until they could return to work (Lyons and Petrucelli, 1978, p. 317).

Emerging from the Dark Ages about 1000 AD, the Middle Ages (through 1500 AD) were Church dominated. Medical education had begun in universities, particularly in southern Italy (Salerno), where diagnoses of somatic disorders and their sequelae were first made. Universities controlled the intellectual life of the elite, and they were usually associated with holy orders. The rich and the poor were still dealt with separately for their ailments. By the twelfth and thirteenth centuries, many of the hospitals that existed were still Church responsibility, but a few were transferred to municipal management. The best (in a manner of speaking) of these were Hotel de Dieu in Paris, Santo Spirito in Rome, and St. Thomas's and St. Bartholomew's in London (Lyons and Petrucelli, 1978, p. 338). However, most were little more than warehouses for the vulnerable. The pattern of care for these hostels remained under Church auspice and support.

The Crusaders were significant in the advancement of hospitals. They cared for their wounded in well-established field hospitals and for those individuals caught in epidemics. However, the Crusaders themselves were responsible for bringing diseases such as typhus, smallpox, bubonic plague, and even leprosy to Europe when they returned. While in the Middle East, they drew on Eastern medicine and also took the prevailing medicines home with them.

In medieval times, medicine was a combination of medicinals and scientific practices. By the Renaissance, in the mid-fifteenth century, while epidemics were rampant, a critical innovation in the form of the printing press fostered medical knowledge. The natural world and the human form could be illustrated, and written materials were used to serve medical education. The scientific revolution followed as studies gave new understanding of diseases, chemistry, drugs, and blood circulation. The microscope and the thermometer advanced knowledge of respiration, the nervous system, and the bone structure. While knowledge was growing by leaps and bounds, the clinical intervention did not change much. Doctors were held both in high regard and also lampooned. Individuals suffering from mental illness were warehoused.

Public health in the seventeenth century in England was appalling for families and children. Unwanted children were simply abandoned to the streets; children of the poor had no access to medical care. The practices in the German states, at the same time, were totally different. German municipalities cared for their citizens and had introduced a form of hospital for care. As feudalism broke down because of the Industrial Revolution, the State became for the first time an important factor in caring for people in need. Large groups of people were uprooted and needed to be assisted. The Elizabethan Poor Law of 1598 created the basis for "poor relief" in England (and subsequently in the United States) and was probably the foundation for all federal law dealing with social and public welfare.

Women served as comforting healers over time—in Egypt, Rome, Greece, Babylon, even in pre-Columbian America. Nursing in the form of caretaking is in evidence from early times. Even before the beginning of the Christian era, nursing was recognized in India. Nursing was not limited to women; men were central in this role during the Crusades, as were priests, particularly in the Middle Ages. Nursing was so closely associated with the church that even a nonreligious nurse was referred to as "sister." When hospitals were no longer church affiliated, the services of nurses and charitable secular women were replaced by the poor as underpaid help who served only the poor—but essentially in maintaining only the housekeeping services. It was not until Florence Nightingale assumed her nursing role in the Crimean war, and reinforced during our Civil War, that nursing became formalized with the introduction of "bedside care." She not only promoted formal education for nurses through lifting them to a respected status, but she also helped to reform military medicine and military medical education (Lyons and Petrucelli, 1978, pp. 543-544). The conditions of war were so appalling that a public hue and cry resulted in establishing the International Red Cross, which set standards for care of the military wounded.

During the nineteenth century, small relief-giving organizations arose in England and on the European continent. As they grew in number, they began to consolidate. By the end of that century, the large Charity Organization Society was established in London. Later, this pattern of social welfare was duplicated in the United States. Private "charities" have always been the forerunners in recognizing social welfare needs and have been responsible for social reform by influencing a state to become active in providing social and health needs.

Lewis Thomas in an article in the *Atlantic Monthly* in April 1981 suggests that therapy is really plain friendship. He recalls that the first recorded therapy, officially titled as such, was performed by Patroclus, referred to by Homer as Achilles' "theragon": "Patroclus was the leader's professional friend." He lived in the same tent as Achilles, listened to his endless complaints, even encouraged him to shout out his anxieties. "He defended and represented his patron against the world, and finally perished in the performance of his duties. Therapy means standing by in steadfast, affectionate and useful companionship" (p. 42).

In one sense the social services* and the social needs and issues and reform in medicine go hand in hand throughout time. The means to "help" others, the "standing by" of Patroclus, is a phenomenon of early times, ranging from self-help, to tribal and/or cult group assistance in the form of shamans, witch doctors, the priesthood, and municipalities—all of whom listened and responded in cultural context. Women were generally in the forefront of giving succor and aid to the needy. If one considers the formal beginning of medical social services, 1636 appears to be the date when Vincent de Paul is anointed as "the patron saint of all hospital social services" (MacKenzie, 1919,

---

* For a discussion of early social services, see "Social Work and Health Care, Yesterday, Today, and Tomorrow" by H. Rehr and G. Rosenberg in *Social Work at the Millennium,* edited by J. G. Hopps and R. Morris (pp. 86-122), The Free Press, New York, 2000.

p. 95). From then until the French Revolution, the hospitals in Paris had recognized social service auxiliaries. The auxilians were mostly women who brought "material and moral aid" to those in the wards, as well as some financial support to the institutions. They made home visits, carrying informed advice to "at home" care. During the French Revolution, the auxiliaries were abandoned, but reestablished again at the Hotel de Dieu, which also served as a hospice for the terminally ill. Auxilians returned to serve in the hospitals in France.

At the London Hospital, Sir William Blizzard set up a comparable organization in 1791 to serve the sick poor. The London Charity Organization Society was created in 1869 to improve the conditions of the poor and to stem mendacity. However, London doctors protested against "free care" for those they believed could and should pay a fee for medical care. In 1874, the Royal Free Hospital sought to introduce "ability to pay" in an attempt to exclude ineligibles. It was Charles Loch who identified the need for a "charity assessor" (the hospital almoner of the future) to deal with financial eligibility for care. Again the poor and those able to pay were separated as to the source of care: the poor went to the Charity Organization Society, and the payers went to the Provident Dispensaries, which were fixed-fee clinics.

The hospital almoner was formally recognized in 1895, stationed at the Royal Free Hospital "to review applicants for admission to the dispensary and to exclude those unsuitable for free care" (Cannon, 1952, p. 25). One of the first functions of social service in hospitals was to serve doctors as financial screening agents to exclude those who could pay for care.

Hospital almoners in England, while screening for eligibility, began to uncover other social needs and environmental problems related to the patients' illnesses. By 1911 the National Health Insurance Act formally endorsed the concept of almoners by broadening their functions to deal with the range of social-health needs of the populace.

The nineteenth century introduced the beginnings of modern medicine in Europe. At the same time, the Industrial Revolution was impacting factory working conditions and social-environmental conditions. Communicable diseases such as cholera and yellow fever were commonplace. Concurrently, scientific societies and the universities were making contributions to medical knowledge. Also the hospitals in Europe began to shift from warehouses to laboratories for learning for physicians. Europe's medical care patterns and the role of auxilians and almoners became the prototype for American medicine but not until the end of the nineteenth and early part of the twentieth centuries.

The credo of a given religion governed who was to receive assistance. Poverty was the key determinant. It was thought the Church would improve the lot of humanity, but the Church was essentially ineffectual. The Industrial Revolution contributed to the breakdown in "social development." Machinery in its contribution to industry became more paramount a concern than humanity. The propertied classes governed the unpropertied (except for the short period of the French Revolution). In general, dictators and the royal houses had no relation to social deprivation. There were periods when individuals rose to challenge the status quo—to relieve the distress of given persons in society. Occasionally small communes set up to deal with inequality with the privileged classes, but unsuccessfully. Socialism and communism were other later forces to deal with social inequalities and injustice.

The history of the social services in medical care is interrelated with the history of medicine. Culture, the supernatural, religion, and tribal rituals as they affected the healing practices on behalf of the sick also affected the aid patterns. Resources and knowledge development move the patterns of social and illness care from self-help in the early times to tribal support, divination and magic, to the priest-physician, religious charity, municipal supports, and by the seventeenth century to a sort of structured but lay social services in hospitals. This means of helping others became recognized, and a formal body of helpers was established by the end of the nineteenth century—the beginning of social work as a profession in the United States.

Chapter 3

American Medicine and the Emergence of the Social Work Profession

INTRODUCTION

As one considers the development of American medicine, the changes from the beginning of the twentieth century are remarkable when viewed in the latter half of the past century and into the beginning of the twenty-first century. There is a different professional and scientific world for medicine as it is for social workers as well. The turning point has been suggested as following World War II (Rogers, 1986). The expectation of medical care for the war's injured became the expectation of the American public. Major social and economic changes, prevailing values, and new knowledge and technology impacted medicine and social work in medical services and in social welfare.

Social work, which was linked to the traditional medical model of care, appeared in hospitals. As social-environmental-psychological determinants were seen as affecting individual's health status, a new social-health approach was initiated as a more comprehensive modality of care. Health care became a political, financial, governmental, and a provider and public issue in regard to health care delivery.

America passed from a "golden age" in medicine (Rogers, 1986) to a new age in this century affecting medical and social-health care priorities. The issues of concern regarding quality, access, and continuity are currently being raised by providers, the public, and society in general.

The history of American medical and nursing care during the eighteenth and nineteenth centuries is glaringly black. It was essentially provincial unlike English medicine, which was "rigidly controlled by guilds and dominated by dogma" (Ebert, 1973). The colonialists in the New World rebelled against "those 3 great scourges of mankind, priests, lawyers and physicians—for the people were too poor to maintain their learned gentlemen" (Ebert, 1973, p. 103). The therapies then were not unlike those in earlier times such as blood purges, enemas, and fumigations (Lyons and Petrucelli, 1978). There was no science to medicine, and its ministrations had little therapeutic benefit.

The expanding American West produced a barbershop frontier type of medical care. Medical institutions as such were proprietary. As the population moved west, there was an unprecedented expansion over enormous territory. Although the need for doctors prevailed, an untrained personnel administered care as sought. If a hospital type of institution did exist, it was staffed by those whose only training was in apprenticeship (Rosner, 1978). Whatever training for medicine existed in the nineteenth century, it was set up by commercial for-profit groups that graduated thousands of doctors with little knowledge and skill. American medicine was essentially based on apprenticeship.

Hospitals were charity hostels for the sick poor. They were essentially poor relief establishments—a town charity. Following the English Poor Law, the American well-to-do created hospitals to keep the dying off the streets and as a means to control disposal of the dead. A few cities such as Philadelphia (in 1751), New York (in 1771), and Boston (in 1811) created hospital–hostels. The federal government set up a Marine Hospital Service to care for sick sailors in port, using a tax on their wages to pay for care. Almshouse infirmaries were poorhouse caretakers and along with hospitals were the training locales for doctors.

In those times, it was not uncommon to see impoverished sick patients cleaning floors and washing linens. In the context of the Darwinian theory "survival of the fittest," they were expected to assist in whatever ways the staff requested. Hospitals were charity social services rather than medical institutions as we know them today. However, a few innovations were promulgated, organized by medical and social leaders in the late nineteenth century influenced by European medicine and a sense of humanitarian beliefs. Some went for training to European universities and hospitals. When they returned to the United States, they brought with them their newfound learning. Science had begun to enter European medicine, where new discoveries, new understandings of disease, and new techniques were developing (Starr, 1980, pp. 37-40). As the twentieth century began, this knowledge was then transferred by returnees to American medical establishments affiliated with universities (Ebert, 1973, p. 103). Medicine's role in the United States was changing from the custodial to the remedial under the drive of these elite institutions.

Their exposure to scientific knowledge led physicians to influence a few institutions: New York Hospital with Columbia University and later Cornell Medical College; Massachusetts General Hospital and Harvard Medical School; Pennsylvania's Hospital and the University; and, in New York City, Bellevue Hospital and its affiliation with the New York Medical School (Knowles, 1973, p. 92).

The all-purpose sick and social service hospital changed as doctors began to turn to the hospital and dispensary to serve as a workshop and laboratory for dealing with illnesses. They began to exclude the long-stay patients, shifting the emphasis to a voluntary medical institution to deal with the acute biomedical care needs of the populous. Flexner's study of existing medical education (1925) with the support of the Carnegie Foundation was the birth of biomedical education and practice in this country. One outcome of his recommendations was the separation of clinical practice from public health care. The changes in hospital shifted the power in leadership from lay to medical. Rosner (1978), however, suggests that the radical change in hospitals from custodial to remedial is due to social factors including the Depression, economic instability, massive immigration, and a general social disorganization at the beginning of the twentieth century (p. 17).

"Whether or not these factors were responsible for change in hospitals, they were certainly responsible for the changing emphasis in social welfare and the social reform movement" (Leiby, 1978, p. 74). Medicine and social work were without an organized base at the beginning of the twentieth century. Although John Hopkins was in the forefront of American medical education, it along with the American Medical Association (created in 1847) via its council on medical education and the Carnegie Foundation for the Advancement of Teaching brought Abraham Flexner to survey the field (1915). He found medicine seriously flawed, and his conclusion resulted in the grading of schools for their quality.

SOCIAL WORK EMERGES

Medical social work in this country has its roots in the 1850s. The forerunners to the medical social work movement were the women doctors who pioneered in medicine. Elizabeth Blackwell, founder of the New York Infirmary for Women and Children, engaged in home visiting of needy patients. She trained mothers in child care and in good housekeeping and sought a social service for the sick poor. Hygiene and health education were encouraged by Anne Daniel (also of the New York Infirmary). She, too, saw a role in motivating her patients to follow medical recommendations by supporting their needs in the home. These doctors were activists in seeking to improve both living and working conditions, which they saw as impacting the health of the poor. They drew on other doctors and volunteers to teach sanitation and diet to their patients. They sent out a "sanitary visitor" whose responsibility was home visits to discharged patients and selected outpatients (Cannon, 1952).

A similar experience to that of the New York Infirmary was that of Dr. Marie Zakrewski. She was a protégé of Dr. Blackwell and as Professor of Obstetrics at a Boston medical college advanced home visits as a medical care follow-up and as a medical educational experience for medical students to understand the impact of social and sanitary conditions.

These were evidence of an early practice of family medicine that dealt with social and environmental factors in illness. The program initiated by Dr. Blackwell moved responsibility for at-home care from doctors to nurses to social workers. Social workers carried home visiting into the beginning of the twentieth century, while in some parts of the country the nursing profession undertook it. Some doctors at the turn of the century thought nurses should carry social service functions and others thought social workers should have nursing training (Cannon, 1952, pp. 25-26).

SOCIAL WORK CONNECTS TO MEDICINE

Social work in medical services in America has had a complex history starting at the turn of the nineteenth century. It has been shaped by political and social events during which it has both gained development and lost ground. The two major wars fought by the United

States strengthened the field of social work when a supportive service for the military was created through governmental and voluntary organizations, via veterans' programs, and in the rehabilitation of those affected by military services. World War II was a most instrumental factor in impacting medical research and services. The responsibility for enhanced medical care of soldiers activated the scientific community (universities et al.) and the government in transforming American medicine (Cluff, 1986, p. 140). Further gains occurred when the federal government recognized the value of the services by payment for care given to those in need. This was evidenced in the legislation that created Medicare, Medicaid, and the maternal and child health, and other health-oriented programs. As funding for hospitals increased, so did the social work services in the institutions. Mandating the availability of social services in hospitals was the formal recognition by the American Medical Association via its Joint Commission on Accreditation of Hospitals (currently JCAHO) in ensuring that services were available to patients and families.

In the mid-1900s, the country was in an industrial revolution, shifting from a rural agrarian state to an urban society. The United States became the immigration haven and the flow of immigrants into the Northeast helped create crowded living slums and appalling factory work conditions. Disease was rampant, with slum dwellers suffering tuberculosis, cholera, typhus, and typhoid fever.

These social and economic problems addressed via the "War on Poverty" contributed to the changing character of medicine, and they certainly affected the social welfare. Welfare as it existed had been largely "custodial rather than remedial" (Rehr, 1982, p. 43). The early approach to assisting individuals was based on "worthiness" and in separating those who were "fit" from the unfit in the community. The objective was the protection of the larger population (Axinn and Levin, 1975). The early beliefs supported the notion that pauperism visited from parent to child. Charity by the well-off was oriented toward teaching the poor morality and the value of work so as to build character.

Social work, as we know it today, had its beginning in the late nineteenth century. The beginnings were a social service that undertook and participated in a number of functions that both church and family (and neighbors) dealt with to meet the needs of those who were most vulnerable. They were (and are) entrenched in a private, voluntary, and philanthropic pattern as a form of "social welfare." The helpers tended to concentrate on individuals (the family) and on specific needs rather than on an overall social welfare program. However, as the helpers began to observe the collective social problems evidenced in groups of people, a social reform movement began. Socially minded civic leaders and doctors became the social reformers, calling for environmental changes and improvements in the human condition (Ebert, 1973, p. 183).

The social services in American hospitals, formally initiated in 1905 at Massachusetts General Hospital, evolved from the work of laywomen who facilitated the development of organized social services (the first department in the country) and nursing, by prodding the male-dominated medical institutions to be responsive to the social needs of the poor. Dr. Richard Cabot is credited with medical social work's initiation at the hospital. However, the charity organization movement, the English hospital almoner, and the women's medical education movement were already in evidence. Cabot's ideas for social services were based also on the work of Dr. Joseph Pratt, who had instituted the "friendly visitor" in 1905 as part of the treatment of tuberculosis patients (Williams, 1950).

> Cabot expanded Pratt's "friendly visitor" into a new concept of professional medical care. Cabot's initial vision of medical social work was far more ambitious than the version that eventually gained acceptance . . . . he saw social work as a near equal partner to physician care, with doctor-directed medical diagnosis and social worker-led social diagnosis complementing each other. (Dodds, 1993, p. 419)

At the end of the nineteenth century and the beginning of the twentieth, physicians such as Adolph Meyer, Richard Cabot, William Osler, Francis Peabody, William Putnam, and Charles Emerson, with nurses and lay leaders, created the After-Care Movement in Psychiatry. The social worker served as the investigator and gatherer of information for these doctors, who functioned with the belief that social and environmental factors were responsible for given diseases. Those beliefs led to the development of home supports in the form of home care and social services to patients and families. These leaders brought to medical education the need to expose their students to the community environment, working conditions, and people's homes to search out the etiology of illnesses. Medical students worked alongside the new medical social service workers as "friendly visitors." The emphasis was on family, the neighborhood, and the workplace. The charity organization and the settlement house movements revealed the vast social and health needs of people living in crowded, deplorable urban conditions. Prevention and improvement of the social-health aspects of individuals surfaced as the means to deal with social problems. (Rehr and Rosenberg, 2000, p. 90)

A social reform movement arose as a result of their observations that was directed at legislative and community levels. The leading social reformers of the era, such as Dorothea Dix, Jane Addams, and Edith Abbott (Rosenberg, 1967, pp. 229-230), together with physicians who held similar beliefs led the movement. Dr. Meyer had already developed the children's health and mental health care program in the creation of the Child Guidance Clinic. The aftercare clinic movement was the creation of leading psychiatrists and charity organizations "to provide aid" to discharged patients from mental hospitals. Social workers were assigned their responsibility (Deutsch, 1946).

While the public's health remained a major concern in the first part of the twentieth century, medicine, and later nursing, shifted their concentration to the clinical in the care of the individual as their primary function, and social-health policy was secondary. Similarly, the social reform movement contributed to social work's separating the clinical and the social welfare. All three professions today continue the separation of clinical and social-health policy. The health care professionals dominate the clinical arena, leaving the public health to others. Social workers in medical settings were not autonomous in their practice. They were frequently directed by bureaucratic or physician-determined expectations. By and large, their work in the early period was not in their control. Social workers, like nurses, frequently were referred to as "handmaidens" to doctors. These two areas remain female dominated in a still male-dominated field. Both have sought autonomy (Ebert, 1973, p. 103). Autonomy in the health care field is dichotomous with both the professional and administrative lay authorities, each seeking to be in control. Autonomy issues, along with interprofessional conflicts, surface over and over in many forms.

"Turf conflicts are still prevalent between doctor and nurse" (Lowe and Herranen, 1981) and between

> doctor and social worker, nurse and social worker, social worker and hospital administrator, and between those dual authorities responsible for institutional service, the medical and the lay boards. Roles and functions of the many health care professionals in the institution have continued to become more confused and overlapping. (Rehr and Rosenberg, 2000, p. 48)

Flexner (1915) in his study of social work identified its many problems. His was an early attempt to formalize a scientific base for its services (Ebert, 1973, p. 104). Mary Richmond (1917) wrote *Social Diagnosis*. Her philosophy was "to define the situation and the personality of an individual with a social need." She encouraged helpers to assist an individual to change and not to do to or for him or her (p. 104). Drawing on her work, medical social workers attempted to relate social diagnosis and medical diagnosis. The American Red Cross was influential in its provision of social services to the military men and their families during World War I. Social workers were drawing on Richmond's philosophy and on those of the early mental health movement and were attempting to integrate "social diagnosis" as an assessment for care. Social and environmental conditions were recognized as contributing to given diseases as well as to social problems. However, in the early 1920s and into the early 1930s, social work moved to accept a psychoanalytic framework for its casework services. The 1929 Depression reintroduced the need for a range of welfare benefits and economic and concrete services. Short-term care dealt with "reality" problems. These philosophical differences—meeting need via a counseling relationship versus the Depression's social welfare trend—have remained conflicting for social work.

In 1929, President Herbert Hoover appointed doctors, public health experts, and social workers as well to the White House Conference for Child Health and Protection. A subcommittee of medical social services contributed to the study of children's health status in 1930 with the objective to contribute to their welfare. The subcommittee functioned under the Section on Medical Services. To further elaborate on the social services of the time, Cannon (1952) noted that of the 6,700 hospitals in the country (public and voluntary; general and specialized), a little over 10 percent (700) had social service programs.

She noted that social services were initiated in a Boston hospital when a physician recognized that a pregnant mother with tuberculosis whom he was treating could not be cared for by medical treatment alone.

The medical social service subcommittee made its report to the White House Conference noting that "human disease and defect are never isolated, but exist always in a complex of personal and environmental conditions. These conditions may favor or hinder recovery, and must therefore, be taken into account in the treatment of sickness of the patient" (Cannon, 1933, p. 13).

In 1928, the American Association of Hospital Social Workers established standards for social service departments, and the American College of Surgeon accepted these. Quality discharge planning for children in particular was reported to the White House Conference as a key function of social service. Cannon also notes that in 1930 social service and nursing were working together to undertake community surveys of medical need. She was already recognizing the link with public health. There was even some evidence of social workers assisting the private patients of given physicians who asked for assistance. This adjunct service was supported at Baker Memorial Hospital Training Centers for social workers, which emphasized medical content. She reported that eleven centers for medical social services existed at that time in hospitals in major cities. The social factors in sickness were also being transmitted by social workers to medical students in a few academic medical centers.

As we noted, in the beginnings of social work in hospitals, medicine was a learned "art" taking place in the wards of charity hospitals—both voluntary and public. A dedicated group of physicians served the poor sick and trained medical students and house staff on these patients. In those days of the 1940s one of the authors made "ward rounds" with physicians. Doctors talked to each other—assessing and educating as they moved from bed to bed. They rarely addressed the patient other than for information. Social workers worked alongside these physicians, learning diagnoses and trying to impact their assessments of patients and their needs—a beginning toward a social-health frame of reference. The medical concern then was "compliance" with their recommendations. Compliance changed to motivation, then to sharing and to partnership between doctor and patient involving diagnostic awareness, its implications, and treatment.

The ambulatory clinics were not much better in the forties. They were gloomy areas where patients waited for voluntary physicians who were ready to see them. Medical care was hands-on diagnosis, which has changed to today's extensive laboratory and technological tests to determine a diagnosis.

Social work services were dominated by psychoanalytic theory from World War I to World War II. By the 1940s, the field entertained a transition to the social sciences, which were beginning to achieve status. As social workers witnessed people's social-environmental and occupational problems and needs, they began a reemphasis of social concern and for social welfare. Nevertheless, individual psychology and its therapy, a "relationship-based" formulation between social worker and client, was prevalent. The major emphasis was on both the inner and outer worlds of the client. Both neighborhood and the community were seen as the loci for services for individuals and groups at risk. At the same time group services and community development efforts were introduced in health care settings, and special health programs were introduced in the community.

The social problems that were most evident in the 1950s were as a result of the proliferation of homeless persons, illegal aliens, and the uninsured sick in major cities. Also an aging population made greater demands on the resources of the health care system. Differences rather than homogeneity as the norm was recognized of people living in communities. Work environments were in flux due to new technologies that affected not only the labor environment but also the workers' health entitlements.

Major life changes had occurred between 1900 and 1960. Life expectancy had risen from forty-seven to seventy years of age. This was due largely to public health measures, improved living conditions, the discovery of "wonder" drugs, and major surgical improvements. The Roosevelt administration created a range of service support programs to assist the unemployed and economically depressed. Roosevelt also projected medical care in the form of a national health insurance program for the American populace in the 1930s. Its passage was unsuccessful due to the opposition of the American Medical Association. Social Security did pass in the Roosevelt administration and was expanded into Medicare and Medicaid and into the Maternal and Child Health Service in 1965. However, note that industry had introduced a form of health insurance (General Motors insured its employees as early as 1928), and the Depression had produced Blue Cross (Cluff, 1986, p. 153).

Midway in the century, in spite of some periodic fiscal concerns, the country entered into a period of affluence, projecting major social service and health care changes. The public was actively invested in the civil rights movement, the women's movement, the drug culture, and the sexual revolution, and more technologic initiatives were introduced than were before. The federal government fostered major advances in the medical and social work fields. Throughout the 1960s we saw The Hill-Burton Act for the construction of hospital beds, an expanded Public Health Service, a burgeoning Veterans Administration, the Health Professions Education Act supporting an expansion of health care providers, Medicare, Medicaid, the Maternal and Child Health Programs, and an active support of biomedical research in the field by the National Institutes of Health. Dr. Howard Rusk had introduced rehabilitation programs for disabled veterans during World War II. One of the results was the development of Physical Medicine for the growing numbers of disabled adults and children. Poliomyelitis, which had been epidemic in the 1950s, was now treated with rehabilitation. Social workers and physicians began to recognize parents as essential in the care of children with chronic illnesses, thus influencing the beginnings of family therapy. Family therapy was also introduced in the care of the mentally ill.

What needs to be recognized are the multitude of advances in medicine in the twentieth century and the extent to which social work in health services has been related to them. The range of medical innovations took various forms:

- the public's health was a major focus of governments and special organizations, which included some social services available to given populations in need and which late in the century becomes a combined public—"social medicine";
- immunology, when fully researched, brought a basic understanding of the immune system; prevention was then projected, but limited funding was available;
- virology brought the understanding of the viral-caused diseases and the availability of vaccines;
- human genetics (genome theory), with its understanding of the genetic factors in diseases, advanced; prevention became signif-

icant; social workers and geneticists competed for counseling roles;
- social work services (both in counseling and in prevention) experienced the impact on patients of genetic disorders (immunology, virology, human genetics) and began to identify a role with both individual and families;
- for cancers, while causation is under constant investigation, social services assumed a very active role in assisting patients and families with the impact of the disease;
- end-of-life decision making, bereavement, and grief therapies are addressed by social work;
- rehabilitation, instituted in World War I and enhanced in World War II, assisted disabled veterans to recover both an optimum physical and social quality of life; rehabilitation became a major social service enterprise; social work was active in counseling and in fostering self-help groups during the poliomyelitis epidemic;
- psychoanalysis, followed by psychotherapy, became the underlying philosophy of social work from World War I until the mid-thirties when a social-environmental psychiatry became more prominent; shock therapy, community psychiatry, behavioral psychiatry, and group therapy followed, with today's emphasis on a biochemical psychiatric therapy.

The latter psychiatric emphasis by social workers tended to separate them from the social workers in the medical arena. However, the current biochemical approach to mental illness appears to bring psychiatry and medicine closer. If that occurs, social work may find its care under an umbrella concept that brings health and mental health together, in service, study, and health maintenance. As one thinks of medicine today—dialysis, transplantation, radiation, surgery, rehabilitation, drug therapy for a range of disorders—it is apparent that a biopsychosocial approach to both diagnosis and treatment with patient and family is critical. A social-health model of care is more comprehensive than is either the traditional medical or psychiatric model of care. By the last twenty years of the century, a social-health model of care had been introduced in most academic medical centers. Social workers were active in this multiprofessional approach to diagnosis and treatment.

The fiscal crisis of the end of the twentieth century (and continuing), along with a taxpayers' revolt, brought on a conservatism resulting in limiting the support of existing social benefits and curbed any changes in social-health policy. The national focus, starting in the 1970s, shifted a governmental commitment for the "right to health care" to a so-called safety net. The net served to cap and limit aspects of medical care, resulting in less service for the most needy (Knowles, 1973, p. 92) and in its way created a system of rationing services.

In the beginning of the twenty-first century the payment of health care services has been constricted. As a result more responsibility falls on the individual. Increased premiums, larger deductibles, cutbacks by the federal government in all its programs, and curtailment of employment-based health benefit programs have resulted in more out-of-pocket costs for everyone. At last report by the Bureau of Statistics (2004), forty-five million Americans are without any insurance or have very limited coverage. Those most affected are those with marginal incomes, people of color, those in uncovered work situations, millions of children of these marginally employed people, the poor elderly, the homeless, and illegal aliens. As medical care benefits are cut or stagnate, affecting the way individuals access services, social work services are also cut by most social-health agencies and by insurers to their covered clients.

Hospitals were affected by the fiscal crisis in the mid-1970s. As government shifted from a per diem reimbursement for a length of stay to the diagnostic-related group (DRG) payment for inpatient services, it reduced the length of hospitalization. DRGs prescribed the length of a hospitalization based on diagnosis. The program also placed a greater emphasis on ambulatory services, and a major result was the development of a multitude of one-day surgical programs. Along with new ambulatory services, the shorter stays meant less filled beds and reduced reimbursements.

By the 1980s, deregulation of health care was introduced. It resulted in a shift from hospitals as a public social utility to a commercialized system. A third tier of care was added to that of the voluntary and public hospitals as for-profit health enterprises entered the marketplace. The traditional charitable cost support that hospitals enjoyed in the reimbursement provided by third-party payers was being reconsidered. Insurance companies were challenging this cost, which was included in their payment patterns. Also, there was evidence that, in the privatization of medical care, a practice of "creaming off" the private or well-insured patients who were generally less sick than the medically indigent was happening. The practice benefited the for-profit hospitals, and created severe fiscal impact on the voluntary and municipal hospitals, which were obligated to care for the seriously and long-term ill patients.

As governments (federal and state) put caps on their reimbursement rates, a "de facto" rationing of care became commonplace. Benefits and services were changed, and beds (and hospitals) were closed as occupancy rates were too low to support their maintenance. When the AIDS epidemic hit the major cities there was a severe shortage of hospital facilities for this population, along with limitations in acute and long-term care. Doctors had begun to exclude Medicare patients as the government introduced cutbacks in reimbursement rates for this population.

Outreach to those in need of medical care was a 1960s' phenomenon. It was a political maneuver emanating from the War on Poverty. It attempted to link community needs with academic medical center care. The medical establishment took on a sort of public health stance. Community medicine was a social-health intervention involving the public to deal with disparities in service availability (Johnson, 1986, p. 163). Doctors were not always enthusiastic about dealing with the community populace. However, the 1960s dealt with a "concept" of the "right to care," which surfaced again in the early nineties and was again defeated by a concept of "a safety net." The community investment brought in both social scientists and social workers to uncover those in need of medical care and to require institutions to provide it. (The 1966 Model Cities Act provided reimbursement for services.)

As the fiscal crisis changed the health care delivery system, social work attempted to find pathways to safeguard the quality of care for the vulnerable. Hospital-based social workers introduced a "high social-risk" screening instrument in order to uncover those in need and so as not to be reliant on other health care providers for referral of those in need. They developed a problem classification system, along with their outcomes, to determine the impact of the services on their clients. A patient opinion and satisfaction tool was created to determine whether services in general and specifically were meeting patients' needs. A patient representative program was put into place to deal with institutional obstacles to service, and a social-health advocacy program assisted individuals to deal with securing their entitlements.

As both programs uncovered problems patients faced, their intent was to learn whether improved performance and programs should be introduced. Social workers began to study their clientele and noted commonalities and differences that led to more and more group approaches and innovative programs. Cultural diversity was evidenced and led to learning the impact of cultural factors on individuals' responses to their illness. Social workers in working side-by-side with physicians and nurses helped to foster multiprofessional care for patients. They introduced a biopsychosocial context by demonstrating its benefits to patients in both their diagnosis and treatment. Collaboration with other health care practitioners reflected a true multiprofessional approach to both diagnosis and treatment with care, becoming a social-health model. Social workers along with the women lay leaders socialized the institution, individualizing care within the growing social-health medium with a host of amenities.

In the past thirty years social work has promoted the concept of social-health care in many medical institutions. Its leadership, frequently moving into administrative positions in medical institutions, has demonstrated the importance of individualizing patient care and of humanizing medical care and socializing the institution (Rosenberg and Clarke, 1987). In helping patients to achieve a positive response to hospitalization, while enhancing a patient-family orientation to care, the medical institution and its providers have observed the value of broadening its focus from a medical model to the more comprehensive social-health model.

However, the crisis affecting the fiscal stability of hospitals has threatened the gains achieved. The way social services are paid in health care compounds the problem of making available needed social services to the hospitalized patient and during his or her aftercare. The academic medical center has been in the driver's seat, advancing medical care and educating doctors. The fiscal crisis has put limitations on its educational and service programs. Specialization was now a physician's practice choice. Social workers became more specialized and began serving in specialty units. Specialization led to fragmentation of care. Social workers found themselves in the role of coordination of care for patients. Other factors continue to affect the provision of social work services in health. These include (1) changes in type of ownership and control of hospitals—the shift to for-profit companies in health care (e.g., surgeons setting up their own hospitals, separating care from the general hospital for paying patients); and (2) horizontal integration—the decline of freestanding institutions and the rise of multi-institutional systems (Starr, 1980, p. 429).

Cost controls were a factor in the 1980s and thereafter except for a few short good fiscal periods. The dependency on filling beds required discharging patients as early as possible. The introduction of payment via DRGs made the discharge planning role for social workers a paramount one.

Health care delivery is in flux again. A fiscal conservatism has affected the government and industry, resulting in institutional crises and provider uncertainties.

When faced with crisis, social workers have been motivated to safeguard the quality and the availability of care. However, today, the health care system is deemed to be in crisis. Will social work rise to deal with health care in the context of today's social and institutional change?

Chapter 4

Mount Sinai Medicine and the Women Who Socialized the Institution

The concept of the Jews' Hospital was initiated in 1852 in New York City by men of that faith who were philanthropists and civic leaders to deal with the growing number of Jewish immigrants and Jewish poor. Their wives were close at hand. The setting opened in 1855, not as a hospital as we know medical centers today, but rather as a custodial home for the needy sick. The home, sponsored by a number of Jewish philanthropists, served as a social service hostel for those who were vulnerable and "at risk" in the community. The custodial home was based on a Judeo-Christian tenet of humanitarianism and charity. In Europe these hostels were administered most frequently by the priesthood or by monks or nuns of various religious orders (see Chapter 2). In this country those who were physically and/or mentally disabled received long-term care—more maintenance than nursing care. It was not uncommon for the very poor, who lacked food and shelter, to be admitted as well (Rosner, 1978).

By the mid-nineteenth century, the United States had moved from being predominantly an agricultural to an urban society. As masses of immigrants flocked to these shores, the Northeast became an overcrowded industrial center. Conditions were appalling, with people seeking work while living in squalor. Tuberculosis was commonplace in both factory workers and in slum dwellers. Housing conditions were primitive, and epidemics of cholera, typhus, and typhoid fever occurred. The times were bad, poverty was everywhere (Rosenberg, 1967), sickness was all too frequent; and the dead were usually left in the street.

These conditions formed the impetus for the leading Jews in New York to create the "benevolent, charitable, and scientific society—to be known as the Jews' Hospital" for the purpose of "medical and surgical aid to persons of the Jewish persuasion and for all purposes appertaining to Hospitals and Dispensaries" (Hirsch and Doherty, 1952). An editorial in the *Harper's Weekly* of May 12, 1869, read,

> It is greatly to the credit of the Jews that their arrangements for taking care of their poor are so thorough that a Jewish beggar is seldom or never seen. Their system of charitable relief is found on the principle of placing the needy in a situation to their living, if they are physically able to do so. Otherwise they are pensioned, put into a hospital, or furnished with such regular relief as may be necessary.

The Jews' Hospital was created by men who perceived the need to care for their own sick. However, it was their wives or the wives of leading citizens who were aware that the sick required more than custodial help. Jewish women were actively involved in social services for the vulnerable in the "hospital." Either they assisted with needed materials and tasks, or their own household help gave services in their name. In 1866, the Jews' Hospital changed its name to The Mount Sinai Hospital, thus removing the sectarian implication. The women organized into a ladies auxiliary of the hospital as early as 1868—a first in a New York institution of this type. The auxiliary was formally organized as a Social Service Auxiliary Board in 1916, changed again to Women's Auxiliary Board, and finally in 1974 became the Mount Sinai Auxiliary Board (Appendix III).

The early general service to the sick and the poor was in the context of welfare rather than remedial. The prevailing philosophy, which was to separate the fit from the unfit, held to the beginning of the twentieth century (Axinn and Levin, 1995). The intent was to protect society from the "unworthy." Pauperism was seen as a condition passed from parent to child. By the turn of the century, a belief in Social Darwinism had become evident. Rugged individualism, along with the importance of the environment and a social morality, had surfaced as the rationale for giving assistance. Charity emphasized both service and work as a means by which the poor could build self-respect and character (Axinn and Levin, 1995, pp. 89-92).

Nineteenth century American medicine was provincial. The American doctor was a product of a "diploma mill," graduating after eight to sixteen weeks of education. Admission to these schools required only the skills of reading and writing. Medical care offered no science and was of limited help. American medicine of the times was haphazard and to be avoided by both rich and poor. Medical care was in its formative stage, and, when needed, most care took place in the home (Starr, 1982).

The early records of the Jews' Hospital indicate the therapies offered were comparable to early practices in Europe—cupping and leeching. However, by the end of the nineteenth century, it became evident that some leaders of the hospital's board of directors and some doctors had been exposed to the scientific work taking place in European universities. The board began to import foreign trained doctors who carved the future direction of the hospital, as well as of American medicine. A few hospitals in the United States had initiated a European type of scientific medicine—New York Hospital and its relationship with Cornell Medical College; Massachusetts General Hospital and Harvard Medical School; and Pennsylvania's Hospital and University (Knowles, 1973). In New York City, there was Bellevue and the University of New York Medical School and The Mount Sinai Hospital.

By the turn of the century, the all-purpose custodial and social service hospital had begun to change. The Mount Sinai medical staff, aware of the beginnings of scientific medicine, turned to the hospital for their workshop and laboratories—becoming biomedical and focusing on acute care. The custodial sick and vulnerable were moved to other settings. There was a shift from the "charity" hostel to the "voluntary" hospital, with the primary leadership becoming medical and with the support of a lay group (which continued to be all male). Rosner (1978) suggests that social forces were primarily responsible for the change to remedial care. In particular, those forces were a depression, economic instability, the massive immigration, the growing labor and capital classes, and a general social disorganization at the turn of the century. However, the growing number of better trained medical practitioners together with the public's dissatisfaction with existing medical practices brought the American Medical Association and the Carnegie Foundation to recruit Abraham Flexner (in 1905) to study the patterns of medical education. The impact of those studies was the birth of biomedical education and the transition to a more scientific approach in medicine. This resulted in the medical model of care, which became the established mode (Rehr, 1982).

As noted, the lay and religious commitment to the sick had been evidenced in early records. Women held unique roles in serving the sick poor and were a primary source of labor. Because of their closeness to patients they were able to observe the social fabric of the hospital and to gain a growing recognition of the basic and social needs of patients. They began to use their awareness to bring certain amenities and personal care for patients into the institution.

Their services were not unlike those of Dr. Elizabeth Blackwell, who has been credited for her social services to the sick poor, and for projecting medical education for women. Because she had been denied admission to serve as a physician in New York hospitals, she created her own dispensary in 1853 to care for women and children (later known as The New York Infirmary for Women and Children). The dispensary served as a training center for women doctors. In 1866 (long before Dr. Richard Cabot, who is credited as the physician who founded hospital-based social services for the needy, began his work), Dr. Blackwell appointed a "sanitary visitor" whose function was to visit both discharged patients in their homes and needy outpatients (Cannon, 1952). Dr. Rebecca Cole was a Negro physician who became a "sanitary visitor," and her work has been described as follows:

> Entering into conversation with the mother or father, she ascertains the various facts relative to the physical condition of the family and children—for continued oversight and instruction on hygienic matters. In succeeding calls, the visitor brings up subjects of ventilation, cleanliness, warmth, food, and clothing, making practical suggestions as they seem to be needed in each case—she sometimes taught them to cook—choose food—with economy—if nuisances found, they have been reported to the proper authorities and speedily removed. Employment has often been found for those who need it, for, though the work is educational rather than benevolent, pressing physical wants must be supplied, before any improvement can be attempted. (Cannon, 1952, pp. 25-26)

At the turn of the nineteenth century, the feminist suffragette movement was a strong force for the acceptance of women into the medical profession. The then traditional values held by women and held by men for women were

- to tend the sick—by nurses and social workers
- to make the soup—meaning to serve and nurture those in need
- to create the goodnesses and the felicities of life.

While feminism was beginning at the end of the nineteenth century, the values were considered important and to be retained. Feminists were intent in translating the values into medical care. They hoped to translate them for the men who still remained the majority in medicine. As women entered medicine it was hoped the values would help to change its practices. Although the number of women who chose medicine during and after World War II declined, by 1960 women did turn to medicine in increasing numbers. Women tended to enter the specialties of pediatrics, psychiatry, and neurology. These were areas in which their sensitivity to family, environment, and occupational impacts was evident in their practice. At the same time, at Mount Sinai the women of the auxiliary board continued to bring their sensitivity to the care of the sick.

THE MOUNT SINAI AUXILIARY BOARD

From the beginning of the Jews' Hospital, women had been providing for unmet needs and extra comforts based on their observations. In their early work, they raised funds for needed equipment, supplies, and support of special programs. They were the first to provide social services in the organization, visiting patients in the hospital and in their homes. They assumed responsibility for what has become the current type of health education to assist patients and families to deal with medical recommendations. They assisted families with money and also with food and clothing. As they moved to assist patients in the hospital and in their homes, they brought a humanistic and social orientation to the institution and to its providers of care (MacEachern, 1940).

Social services grew out of the efforts of these lay women who encouraged the development of organized social services and nursing by urging their male partners to act on behalf of the social needs of patients and to humanize the institution. The Mount Sinai women have been involved from the beginning. As noted, a ladies auxiliary was recognized by the board of trustees in 1868. From a Committee on Social Welfare initiated in 1911, a Social Service Auxiliary Board was formally created in 1916 setting as its objective "to supplement the medical care provided by the Hospital by such services as will further the welfare of the patient and his family" (Stein, 1953, p. 46). Today, the members are a group of thirty-four dedicated volunteers committed to the enhancement of patient care.

The women's efforts along with the farsightedness of the medical and other lay leaders of the institution led to the creation of a philanthropically supported social welfare department in 1906. In 1908, the hospital endorsed a permanent budgetary allocation for the support of social services, noting,

> It is now recognized that the condition of a patient's family while he is on the wards, as well as his needs immediately after his discharge from the hospital, constitute so vital a part of his ability to recover, and to retain his health, that the work of this department has come to be recognized as a legitimate part of the functions of this institution. (Hirsch and Doherty, 1952, p. 151)

In 1974, the Mount Sinai Social Service Auxiliary of 1916 became the Mount Sinai Auxiliary Board, serving as a joint committee of the boards and of the School of Medicine. In 1954, in recognition of the work of the auxiliary board, the then board of trustees appointed the auxiliary board president to trustee membership pro tem. The practice of pro tem appointment continues. Over time a few women have been elected to trusteeship on their own merits. The auxiliary board constituted a corps of women (some men joined) serving as volunteers to further the "general welfare of the patient and family by complementing the hospital's clinical activities with a variety of social and auxiliary services."

The roles assumed by the Mount Sinai Auxiliary Board have been twofold:

1. advocacy
   a. within the institution in recognition of the need to individualize patient care and to bring socialization and amenities to enhance the quality of care;
   b. in recognition of community social-health needs so as to affect public policy for the enhancement of medical and social services for local residents and others;

2. program development by providing seed money for the support of enhanced services for patients as projected by health care providers and by serving as liaison with other institutional personnel in the implementation of such programs.

From the inception of the formal Social Service Auxiliary, with Mrs. Herbert Lehman as its first chairperson and with members drawn from families whose history was lodged in Jewish philanthropy, the members worked as volunteers, reporting needs both from their observations based on volunteer assignments and from informed studies (see Appendix VI). Conscious of the social conditions and of the gaps in the hospital services, generations of dedicated volunteers have viewed patient care as their primary focus, together with recognition of the social needs of the residents of the community. Funds were made available from bequests and from the auxiliary board and friends for their use for patients' needs and to enhance services by demonstration projects and by education. People responded by giving funds for social-health projects within the institution and by increasing the social service staff as need was demonstrated.

Their investment in the changes in the institution was furthered as professional social work was introduced in 1953. The volunteers assisted in the creation of new programs by working closely with the social service department, which the auxiliary helped to create, and in forming linkages with community-based social service programs. From the early involvement of the auxiliary board with the hospital, the socialization of the institution and the creation of its social amenities and innovative projects were due to its efforts (see Appendix V). Members created a department of volunteers and introduced occupational recreational therapy, a patients' library, a play school and kindergarten, a workshop for job training, and a sheltered workshop for the disabled. A gift shop was created in the community, known as the "Green Box," for marketing of the sheltered workshop products to produce income for the institution. The Mount Sinai Auxiliary Board initiated a rehabilitation program, supported convalescent and camp care, and gave financial support for individual needs (see Appendix V).

The institution staff submits requests for projects to assist patients and to create innovative services, which are reviewed by the auxiliary's project funding and review committee. Innovative projects frequently find auxiliary members working with the professional staff to achieve the objective. Some of these projects have been finding posthospital housing for discharged psychiatric patients, establishing a CPR training program, establishing and staffing the surgical patients' family waiting room, and providing preadmission telephone outreach to the elderly about their posthospital needs.

The auxiliary has also been responsive to the social conditions of local and national concern. In its work at the beginning of the twentieth century, it responded with offering special services to the vast number of immigrants who flooded New York City and to the many who turned to the hospital for medical care. When an exposé of East Harlem's children revealed the number of them with eye problems, the board supported an eye screening program for children in the schools and subsequently met the needs of those children by providing health education classes and/or treatment. A study revealed an uncovered number of East Harlem residents who had sickle cell disease. The board supported a multidisciplinary team to deal with these patients and their families. The Secondary Education Through Health Program (SETH) was initially supported by the auxiliary before it was supported by state funding. That program was designed to expose East Harlem high school students through courses and hands-on experience at Mount Sinai to health care. The SETH students demonstrated the best attendance records in school, and 90 percent went on to college. Aftercare for the discharged hospitalized patient is also an area that the auxiliary board responded to when it was demonstrated by social workers to be a critical need of patients. To this end the board has supported a home care social worker—following the tradition set by the ladies auxiliary in the nineteenth century.

The auxiliary board initiates projects that are directed at patient care and that have been the result of its support of either social work or interprofessional studies of patient needs. The members were responsible for initial support of the Patient Representative Program, which assists patients in dealing with difficulties and complaints with service, of the Spinal Cord Project, a Comprehensive Breast Service, the Resource Entitlement and Advocacy Program (REAP), a waiting room for the families of surgical patients, and an Employee Assistance Program (EAP). A Department of Health Education was initiated, offering health promotion services for older adults who are patients living in the hospital area; the Family Resource Center Library provides print and audiovisual materials for diversion to patients while hospitalized, and as educational material to help patients and children cope with maternal/child health issues, including wellness and health promotion.

The auxiliary board also assisted in the creation of the hospital's Caregivers and Professional Partnership (CAPP), which trains and supports family caregivers of patients who have returned home but with physical and/or social limitations. Among its recent supported programs is the Pet-Assisted Therapy Program, which promotes patient healing via direct animal-patient interaction. Family violence prevention has been introduced as an educational tool for alerting health care professionals to the risks and to strategies for prevention. Other programs that the board has helped to initiate are Juvenile Diabetes Teaching Service, Holocaust Survivors Project, Palliative Care Project, a Pain Management Program, Methadone Maintenance, a Hospital Corps and Visitors Guide, and Communicard (to assist non-English speaking patients in their medical care). The board has underwritten group therapy programs for Holocaust survivors, stroke patients, speech disorder patients, teenaged mothers, and parents of babies at risk.

The auxiliary board has a commitment to the needs of the East Harlem residents. The group has developed a special social service prevention and health care program for this community's children, a Mom Program, and Mom and Tots Program for local pregnant and parenting adolescents, and an outreach program to parents of premature and seriously ill children.

The auxiliary board is involved in public health policy issues related to patient care delivery and to the changing health care environment. It is committed to the varied communities the institution serves. It contributed to the support of the Center for Multicultural and Community Affairs. It also supports the Health Careers Pipeline Mentoring Program, which opens the door to youngsters interested in entering the health care field. The board, through its legislative committee, has carried its social action concerns beyond the hospital walls. Its social activism includes lobbying in state and federal legislative halls on behalf of social-health policy issues, as well as on housing and employment needs. The board supported an educational program for legislative aides to state and federal officials in learning about academic health science centers and local community needs.

Conscious of the evolving needs of the hospital's patients and of its communities, the board is committed to enhancing the education of health care providers. It provided major gifts to the capital campaign of the hospital and the medical school. It supports awards to outstanding medical students and to social workers for excellence in practice and to those who have made contributions to the hospital and/or patient care. In addition, it supports special health education and information events, conferences, and seminars.

Much of what the auxiliary board seeds in the way of projects is done through its relationship with the Department of Social Work Services and with the service departments of the medical center. It has supported the development of the Hunter College School of Social Work–Mount Sinai Consortium to enhance social work education via an academic-practitioner model. The book describing the experience has served to change social work education across the country (Caroff and Rehr, 1985). An interprofessional education project exists to promote the value of multiprofessional collaboration in diagnosis and treatment. Jeanette Regensberg's study of the interprofessional experiences of social work and medicine was published in 1978. All of these were with the support of the Auxiliary. The department, with support, developed a research program of its services and its information system and a quality and quantity evaluation system. The lay and professional linkage has always underpinned the commitment of the Auxiliary Board.

SUMMARY

From the beginning of the Jews' Hospital, women have been present in the socialization of the institution, in the support of the social-health needs of the hospital's community of patients, and in the support of access to and quality of care. The male-dominated medical institution has shifted from being a conventional medical model of care to having a more social-health orientation. The times have brought more women into medicine (50 percent of Mount Sinai's Medical School admission class). The women medical students do bring something different into their education. As noted, the board of trustees has recognized the women's contributions to both the hospital and the medical school by electing a number of women to trusteeship, while the current president of the auxiliary board holds ex-officio trustee membership.

In addition, the board of trustees has formalized the position of the community board (see Chapter 8) by assignment of one of its members. The women of the auxiliary board and those on the board of trustees bring a dimension that focuses on the comprehensiveness and the quality of care—as they would want it for themselves and their families. The women's investment at Mount Sinai (both Auxiliary members and social workers) has been, in a subtle way, a challenge to the conventional medical model. The women's voice, representing the consumer of care, has been a voice for change. By focusing on the health and welfare of children, families, and the community, they have been in the forefront of facilitating the development of a social-health model of care.

It continues to be the women, both of the auxiliary board and in the social work services, who fulfill the mission of the hospital. They value the medical and scientific innovations the professional staff has introduced in the institution. They also have understood the risks, needs, impediments, and barriers that affect the quality of health care. They have from their beginnings with the Jews' Hospital enhanced the hospital's provision of care and the medical school's education of the men and women for tomorrow's social-health oriented practice of medicine.

The women of the auxiliary board have had a profound impact on The Mount Sinai Hospital by providing a humane broad-based social perspective on behalf of patients and the organization. They created new programs, raised important questions, and in the last half of the twentieth century gained status as members of the board of trustees of the Mount Sinai Medical Center. In many ways they are examples of the feminist traditions of the nineteenth and twentieth centuries. They are examples of the pattern of the nineteenth century, when middle- and upper-class women did not focus only on the family, but instead entered civil society to address the problems created by industrialization. They formed social reform movements, built institutions to pursue a social justice agenda, and demanded that the government take an active role in solving the public social problems (Snyder, 2004). In health care, the movement for reform originated not with doctors, but among upper-class women, who had taken on the role of guardians of a new hygienic order. In New York, the impetus came from women in the States Charities Aid Association, who in 1872 formed a committee to monitor the conduct of public hospitals and almshouses. They represented, in the association's own humble words, "the best class of citizens as regards enlightened views, wise benevolence, experience wealth, influence, and social position" (Starr, 1982, p. 155).

Furthermore, though some doctors approved of the ladies' desire to establish a nurses' training school, which would attract the "wholesome" daughters of the middle class, other medical men were opposed. Plainly threatened by the prospect, they objected that educated nurses would not do as they were told—a remarkable comment on the status anxieties of nineteenth-century physicians. When resisted, as they were at Bellevue in efforts to install nurses on the maternity wards, they went over the heads of the doctors to men of their own class who held greater power and authority in the board rooms.

By initiating a social work department as early as 1906, and in 1953 supporting its professionalization, the auxiliary board enhanced the status of social-health services within the institution. It endorsed a biopsychosocial perspective as a necessity in the diagnosis and treatment of patients and the benefits of care when services include a patient and family focus.

The women who were the new social case workers faced daunting conditions. They were employed in service organizations controlled by businessmen as board members and in particular by a board president, who was often the largest financial contributor. Many of the women who served on lay boards completed graduate social work education and had careers as social workers. Social work was and has been largely a "women's" career. However, a number of men have completed graduate studies and entered the field of social work, joining the professional women social workers.

In 1953 De Beauvoir published her book *The Second Sex* in the United States, and Claire Booth Luce was appointed ambassador to Italy, the first woman to be appointed to a major diplomatic office. Also in 1953, Oveta Culp Hobby was appointed as the first Secretary of Health Education and Welfare, and Eleanor Roosevelt publicly allied herself with the Equal Rights Amendment favoring complete gender quality. The women of the Mount Sinai Hospital Auxiliary Board were leaders of their generation and part of the generations of women that formed the progressive core of American society.

The auxiliary board has been and continues to be an integral component of the Mount Sinai Medical Center. Its contributions to the socialization of the institution and its support of the social-health needs of the hospital's community of patients, and of its providers, continue to be impressive, meaningful, and significant. From its inception, the sole mission of the auxiliary board has been to ensure a high quality of social-health services for patients, families, and the community at large.

Chapter 5

Social Work Activist-Leaders: The Making of a Social Work Department

The Social Work Department of The Mount Sinai Hospital has, on local, national, and international levels, been recognized for its contributions. The progress made from its beginnings in 1906 to the end of the twentieth century has been documented (Rehr, Rosenberg, and Blumenfeld, 1998). The department grew from a single social worker to a complement of 180 full-time employees in 2003. The development of social work followed the development of the remarkable scientific and medical innovations achieved by the institution's professionals (Aufses and Niss, 2002). In addition, as Mount Sinai created its medical school within City University of New York in 1966, it recognized the contributions of social work to health care by incorporating a division of social work into the Department of Community Medicine. The department's role in the education of social workers via its academic/practice model with Hunter College School of Social Work was also extended to a role in the education of medical students (Rehr and Caroff, 1986).

The Mount Sinai's Department of Social Work Service was initiated by the women activists who had made their mark in socializing the hospital with humanitarian services to those in need (see Chapter 4). Their menfolk had engaged in a major charitable contribution in the creation of the hospital (hostel) in 1848 for impoverished, sick Jews. The women fostered the individualization of patient care by becoming invested in the hospital's patients and their families. That social activism was furthered by the leaders those women selected to develop a social work department.

BACKGROUND

Structured social services at The Mount Sinai Hospital began in 1906 when the board of directors of the hospital established a social welfare department. This was among the earliest of such hospital departments in this country. Mount Sinai's social services followed the pioneer program established at Massachusetts General Hospital in Boston and that of Bellevue Hospital in 1906 as the second or the third, depending on who reports it. The initial services were offered by a graduate nurse, Jennie Greenthal, appointed by the Director of the Hospital, Dr. S. S. Goldwater, whose social and public health commitments in health education for the poor in the community have been reported (Aufses and Niss, 2002, p. 13). Dr. Goldwater's assignment to Ms. Greenthal was that she offer discharged patients from the wards information regarding convalescent care, their medical needs, and any employment opportunities available. Soon Ms. Greenthal expanded activities to include home visits to give patients advice, and instruct mothers of newborns in the care of children; needed clothing and carfare and medical supplies were made available. Referrals were also made to convalescent homes and to local relief societies. As the demand for services increased, Ms. Rose Johnson, headworker from 1908 to 1915, urged the members of the auxiliary board's social welfare committee to augment the staff. More nurses were appointed to meet social service needs as the institution created new clinics such as the Children's Health Club, the Mental Health Clinic, Occupational Therapy, general medical clinics, the medical wards, and some specialty services, e.g., Metabolism Clinic.

In 1919 a Children's Health Clinic was established to foster health maintenance and prevention. That service eventually evolved into a behavior clinic supported by a psychologist and kindergartner. In 1920, an adult mental health clinic was separated from neurology, and a social worker was assigned. That service expanded almost every year, finally resulting in the hospital's psychiatric program, with a complement of social workers for each major program.

By the early 1920s, the department was already collaborating with medical interns about the social services offered to their patients. Social histories were affixed to medical charts. Social workers were included in medical rounds, and patients who were planning discharge against medical advice were under 100 percent social service review.

Shelter care for children of hospitalized mothers, hygiene education, re-admission reviews, social agency networking, convalescent care, temporary financial assistance, and nourishment and medical appliances were some of the customary provisions of the social service department. Surveys were undertaken to inform the staff of special situations such as the disposition of neurological cases, the need for convalescent care, the benefits of summer care for children, and the tuberculosis patients who did not show for care. Social services at Mount Sinai were reflective of the prevailing practices of the times. The funding support for the social services in those early years was garnered to a limited extent by members of the board of trustees and by the Federation of Jewish Philanthropy. However, the major source of funds came largely from the members of the Social Service Auxiliary Board, who also managed to secure the in-kind needs that this department required for its clientele.

In 1927, Dr. George Baehr, a leading Mount Sinai and internationally recognized physician, recorded*:

> During the last ten years, Social Service has become one of our most important departments, on a par with medical and administrative services of the Hospital.
>
> Those of us who began our activities at The Mount Sinai Hospital thirty years ago realize that the steady growth of the Social Service Department has been the result of the increasing recognition of the fact that the provision of medical care is only one of the functions of the Hospital, and that medical care cannot be delivered without an equally rational concern for the welfare of the patient and his family, and for those environmental circumstances which may play an important role in the causation or prolongation of illness. An equally important function of the Social Service Department is to keep those human qualities of hospital service, a kindly and thoughtful concern for the patient's future, before the eyes of our physicians, nurses and administrative officials.
>
> Without the reminder of the social service worker, physicians are apt to concentrate their whole activities upon the medical

---

*Foreword, George Baehr, MD, Social Services Department, *The Mount Sinai Hospital of the City of New York: A Review,* 1927-1937 (unpublished report, 1937).

problems of the sick in the wards and to ignore the social problems related to illness which are often equally important to the patient. (p. 1)

In 1923, Mrs. Fannie Mendelsohn (née Lissauer) was appointed headworker (changed to director). Under her leadership, the department continued to expand as its work with patients and their families gained recognition by the board of trustees, knowledgeable physicians, and the women of the auxiliary board. The mission enunciated at that time was that the primary aim of medical social service is to make it possible for every patient to carry out prescribed medical treatment. That mission translated to function and was pursued by the social workers in the 1920s, and supported by the auxiliary board. The workers were expected to add to charts the social histories of their patients, describing them as individuals in a family context and in the community at large. A physical and mental assessment of the patient was shared with the doctor of record. Even in that period, a department bulletin was created and distributed to alert the staff to department, hospital, and community developments.

The 1927 annual report noted that there were thirty-one staff workers, including the director and an assistant director-worker. They covered the following services: medical, surgical, gynecology and neurology, children's cardiac clinic, a children's health class, a luetic clinic, a metabolism clinic, and tuberculosis, cardiac, orthopedic, and mental health clinics. Of the staff, five specialists were designated to cover the following selected units of service: two covered a combined occupational and mental health class, a psychologist covered the children's social services, a kindergartner covered the therapeutic kindergarten and children's health class, and a special surveyor covered the children's cardiac clinic.

An early concern regarding the quality and quantity of the medical social worker's functions appeared in the 1927 report:

> Medical social service on the wards has not yet reached as satisfactory a development as we should like to see. Considerable time is consumed in arranging for the discharge of patients and their after-care, thus not allowing sufficient opportunity to attend adequately to the many other social problems. . . . In order to do the really intensive work needed, the workers should have a small case load.

Listed as some of the activities carried by the department in that period were the following:

1. making hospital care possible by removing personal difficulties;
2. interviewing patients in the wards and outpatient department to ascertain their social needs and presenting such information to the physician that may have particular relationship to the patient and his care;
3. procuring temporary shelter for children whose mothers are ill in the hospital;
4. interpretation of disease and treatment to patients, families, or others interested;
5. educating patients and their families in hygiene;
6. lessening the incidence of readmission of patients through instruction and care supervision;
7. cooperating with other philanthropic agencies; using their facilities and giving them such service as the hospital offers;
8. advising patients in many personal and family problems;
9. arranging for convalescent care in the patient's home or outside of the home;
10. adjusting or securing proper employment;
11. arranging permanent care for the chronic sick;
12. country outings for children during the summer months;
13. providing temporary financial assistance;
14. providing special nourishment; and
15. procuring medical appliances. (Mount Sinai Hospital Social Service, 1927, unpublished report)

The 1927 report concludes by noting that while some of these activities are no longer considered appropriate for the social service department and presently are no longer carried by the department, most of the activities have stood the test of time and experience and remain as important activities of the department.*

---

*The early history of the Social Services at Mount Sinai derives from an unpublished report of the Social Service Department of the Mount Sinai Hospital of the City of New York, 1927 (Archives), and from *Review of Structure, Organization and Functions of the Social Service Department,* The Mount Sinai Hospital, New York City, by Celia R. Moss, 1952 (unpublished report).

One notes some changes in basic philosophy about the function of the social worker in the 1927 annual report. The philosophy and aim of the department was then amended "to make it possible for every patient to carry out the prescribed medical treatment" so that the issue of "compliance or adherence" with a medical recommendation and/or an individual's ability to deal with prescribed care is addressed.

A manual of social services was created for the orientation of staff, along with how to record to medical charts. Medical interns and staff nurses received orientation to social work functions to both inform them about their patients and to alert them to why patients should be referred for social services. Surveys had been undertaken in the 1920s regarding selected populations in need. Although it was recommended to continue surveys to those in need, the lack of funding was a deterrent, and no further study of the social work clientele was undertaken for more than twenty-five years.

By 1937, the social service department had grown to a staff of fifty-four members including professional and clerical staff. Mrs. Mendelsohn was reporting to the hospital's administrator, to the attending medical staff, and to the social service auxiliary of the board. The department offered services to all patients in the children's and adult clinics; supervised the kindergarten, occupational therapy, an exercise class, the workshop to retrain the unemployed, a psychological testing program, and a cadre of volunteers; and created a lending library for patients and staff.

By 1937, the department reported having been involved in more than 14,000 cases involving patients and other health care providers in the hospital. The staff also made more than 13,000 home visits to patient/families to assist in posthospital care. Social work staff education included orientation and continuing "tutorial" conferences which were subject related; and an educational program on the social problems in illness for student nurses in what was then Mount Sinai's Nurses Training School was in place and included not only lectures but field work assessment in the department.

In 1952, a review of the department revealed a lack of core functions and inconsistencies in the performance of social workers in the different services. Recommendations were made to strengthen the relationship with the medical staff and to move to a referral system for those in need, as well as to develop a social service case finding system. Physician contact in all social work cases was mandatory. Although social workers still undertook a financial eligibility review for admission to the hospital, they also drew on admission information as an intake case-finding screening tool. Recording to medical charts was expected, and an educational program was promoted for how to write social service chart entries. Some statistical data reporting in regard to services delivered was also implemented. A recommendation was made to create an avenue for the social service director to contribute to the hospital's policy formulation. Liaison with community social agencies was encouraged, and both social workers and members of the auxiliary board formed committees to accomplish networking to enhance services for community residents.

In 1952, the recommendation was made to the auxiliary board for a professionally trained social work department staff. The recommendation was made by Mrs. Fannie Mendelsohn, the department's director since 1923, and was drawn, in part, from the standards being developed by the American Association of Medical Social Workers. Mrs. Mendelsohn with the support of the auxiliary board was responsible for the growth of the department and expanded social service functions. The professionalization of Mount Sinai's Social Work Service was her retirement wish. The recommendation was supported, and the board brought Celia Moss as consultant to review the department. She projected a professional department based on standards set for social service departments by the American Association of Medical Social Workers in 1949.

The recommendations of that study resulted in the auxiliary board's move with the endorsement of the board of trustees to create a professional social work department to include:

- the director, a recognized professionally accredited master's degree social worker;
- a unified, centralized professional department;
- a social work service accountable to the hospital administration, the board of trustees, and the public it serves;
- an ongoing advisory and supportive relationship with the auxiliary board; and
- expansion of social services to all, based on need.

In late 1953, Doris Siegel, MSW, a consultant with the U. S. Children's Bureau and president of the then American Association of

Medical Social Workers, came to Mount Sinai as director of the department. When Doris Siegel was appointed in 1953, there were four remaining staff members: Anna Levinson (1919), Betty Janover (1919), Pauline Leplin (1926), and Frances Spiegel (1923), who was then the chief social worker in psychiatry. The department had a few support staff, in particular Matilda Markowitz. Mrs. Alfred J. Cook was the president of the auxiliary board.

Under Ms. Siegel's leadership, the department expanded its services and planned and implemented new hospital-based programs for patient care. She did so by uniting all social work services under a centralized professional leadership that supported accountability for service, program study and evaluation, and social work education for the field and for the enhanced practice of the staff. Her philosophy for hospital-based social work services supported a social-health model of care for those who were vulnerable.

In the 1950s, medicine was practiced essentially with a biological and anatomical focus, and social work was on the fringe of the medical practice of its institutions and practitioners. The philosophy enunciated by Dr. George Baehr for a comprehensive biosocial environmental approach to medical care had been lost. Ms. Siegel's social work tenet in that period was to emphasize the need to orient institutional administrators and health care professionals to the biopsychosocial components in diagnosis and treatment of the sick. The social work staff was to demonstrate that those suffering from chronic illnesses needed more than medical advice; they also needed a comprehensive, coordinated, continuum of care. The polio epidemic of that time clearly demonstrated the need to assist these victims with a rehabilitation that included not only physical but also psychological and social supports toward helping patients achieve optimum gains (Sweet and White, 1961). Drawing on Ms. Siegel's visionary plans for social-health care, the department used social work experiences with patients suffering from chronic illnesses and the impact on family life to influence the medical institution to move from a traditional medical model to a comprehensive social-health care model. Social work demonstrated that a biopsychosocial and environmental approach to medical care contributed to both diagnosis and treatment. Social services were designed to motivate patients to follow treatment and to help families to assist patients in dealing with the recovery of physical and social functioning. Family therapy and support groups for patients were instituted, along with community resource networking to offer continued services in the home.

Over a period of almost fifty years into the twentieth century, the department developed and grew, refocusing its mission and roles in the institution in relation to societal and institutional changes (see Appendix I). It provided social services to inpatients and to those in ambulatory care, as well as to residents in the community. In the latter half of the twentieth century, it further expanded under the leadership of four directors (see Appendix I).

The range of social work services at Mount Sinai is vast; it extends to all patient age groups and to almost every medical problem. The social workers have been a vital part of a team of health care professionals that include doctors, nurses, administrators, and others—all of whom work toward providing quality social-health care. In addition to serving those patients and their families known to the inpatient and outpatient services, a major goal of the department was to foster the development of a social-health model of care to override the earlier traditional medical model. In the course of fifty years and into the twenty-first century, under the succeeding leadership of Drs. Helen Rehr, Gary Rosenberg, and currently Susan Blumenfield, the department added to its service commitments:

- a cadre of social-health advocates, an indigenous personnel from the East Harlem community to work with that clientele;
- a corps of patient representatives to serve as institutional ombudsmen dealing with patient-encountered obstacles to care;
- a high social-risk screening means to uncover patients with psychosocial needs both before and at admission;
- information database of social service clientele;
- a social service technician program consisting of aides trained to deal with the defined direct and indirect social services for patients, e.g., finding nursing homes and making transportation arrangements;
- patient satisfaction/opinion surveys as tools for hospital enhancement of services;
- classification of social-health patient problems and their outcome as study means;
- problem identification (the classification system) allowed for the introduction of mutual contracting for services within a patient-client partnership;

- practice-based studies investing the staff in the doing and in the feedback of findings for their practice and program enhancement, with establishment of the Murray M. Rosenberg Applied Social Work Research Center;
- a social-health curriculum for the Brookdale Center for Continuing Education at Mount Sinai for advanced education of practitioners, social workers, students, and other health care professionals;
- a model of an academic-practice partnership of the Hunter College–Mount Sinai Social Work Consortium, which served to offer a theory and an field teaching experience for the enhancement of social work student education (see Rehr and Caroff, 1986);
- the appointment of the Director of Social Work Services as a member of the Hospital's Medical Board, which institutionalized Dr. George Baehr's commitment to a comprehensive service;
- a social work unit in the psychiatric emergency area to triage patients for assignment of needed services;
- the International Enhancement of Social Work Leadership Program at Mount Sinai created for and with Israeli and Australian social work leaders (see *Social Work in Health Care*, 18 [3/4], 1993);
- a founder member of the International Conference of Social Work in Health and Mental Health;
- community liaison via the Model Cities Program and a participant in community programs to further a community-institutional partnership in community health care needs, creating a Community Affairs Division under Dr. Rosenberg and subsequently responsible to the hospital administration;
- founder of and ongoing member in the Medical Center's Community Board;
- the introduction of group and family counseling programs (disease specific, motivationally based, patient-family based);
- served as a consultant to the legislative committee of the Auxiliary Board; created a government relations function for the hospital and medical school;
- continued to staff the auxiliary board, with an emphasis on social-health policy issues as well as the social-health services of the institution;

- created a survey center to measure patient, staff, and faculty satisfaction studies to measure progress in patient care excellence and in human resource improvement programs (these efforts were led by social workers responsible to Dr. Rosenberg);
- a Department of Organization, Change, and Learning established with social workers in the top leadership positions;
- undertook evaluation and applied social work studies, including multiprofessional assessments of care (see Epstein and Blumenfield, 2001);
- engaged in professional accountability for services to patients, the institution, and regulators for quality improvement of social work services and institutional services (see Rehr, 1979);
- enhanced discharge planning services with a continuity of care focus in joint networking with community social agencies;
- engaged with selected community social agencies in the development of consumer health education; developed social work journalism for health education in multimedia; created a unit to deal with promulgating community health education;
- served in administrative roles within the institution, e.g., assistant director, program director, hospital and medical center administrators, department head, etc., and created a unit designed to foster organizational change to lead to better worker morale and organizational effectiveness;
- enhanced the social work role in key services in addition to the primary service areas such as
  —adolescent health care
  —renal dialysis and transplant
  —Holocaust survival
  —pediatric pulmonary care
  —breast and other cancer units
  —myasthenia gravis unit
  —caregivers and professional partnership
  —resource, entitlement, and advocacy program
  —patient representative service
  —amyotrophic lateral sclerosis center
  —hemophilia unit
  —geriatric and adult development unit
  —internal medicine associates
  —palliative care

—child abuse
—substance abuse
—teenage pregnancy
—abortion unit
—sexual assault, violence, and elder abuse

The roles the institution assigned to the social work department, as the needs for given services were demonstrated, led to an active community relationship on behalf of the hospital, to innovative program development, to the development and oversight of the institution's patient opinion surveys of social-health care, and to the development of a community health education program. The department became an advocate along with the auxiliary board to deal with issues of governmental health care programs.

The director of the department carried out these functions and reported to the hospital administrator. The director was a member of the medical board and the community board and helped staff the auxiliary board. The director also delegated key staff to membership on institutional committees and to hospital liaison membership in community agencies.

In 1951, the department joined with the then New York School of Social Work (subsequently Columbia University's School of Social Work) to create a field unit for social work students. The social work department has sustained an educational responsibility for the continued enhancement of its staff practice. It has also from the early 1950s assumed a partnership role with schools of social work in preparing for tomorrow's social work. An academic-practice partnership (a consortium of one school and several Mount Sinai affiliated settings) created a model of social work education to prepare students for effective service in health and mental health settings (Rehr and Caroff, 1986). A member of the staff served as liaison to the curriculum development committee of one of the schools of social work.

When the Mount Sinai Medical School was created in 1965, a division of social work was developed within the department of community medicine. An endowed professorship, the Edith J. Baerwald Professor in Community Medicine (Social Work), the first of its kind in a medical school was created by Jane and Jack Aron, Mount Sinai board members and longtime supporters of quality medical care and social services (see Chapter 8).

The division has been responsible, with the support of the department's social work staff, for a range of academic functions, including its educational programs for health care providers (students and practitioners) and its research enterprises (see Chapter 7).

It is important to cite the department's engagement in assuming a cost-effective accountability for its services. It undertakes quality/quantity evaluative reviews that are reported to administration, the regulators, the payers, and to the clientele, as well as to the staff. The department enhanced its study repertoire to uncover needs and institutional programs and department change.

An illustration of an early study (in the sixties) of elderly users of the institution demonstrated that psychosocial needs were evidenced across class lines (Berkman and Rehr, 1966). Drawing on the consultation of Ruth Fizdale, who created the Arthur Lehman Counseling Service (ALCS), the first not-for-profit social service, Drs. Rehr and Rosenberg established a fee for social services based on an overtime hourly commitment of staff to serve patients, not only discharged patients, but also the private office patients of the hospital's attending staff. The fee-for-social services continues today, producing revenue for the department.

The department enjoyed leadership in its work in assessing early access to social services and in its pioneering studies of referral patterns of patients and families to social services. In uncovering the gaps in reaching those in need, the department developed high social-risk screening techniques, assessing early access to care for those in need. Social-risk screening became one of the major quality of care expectations supported and accredited by the Joint Commission of Accreditation of Health Organizations (JCAHO). Social-risk screening made social work responsible for its own case-finding.

The work in accountability, program evaluation, and staff studies of their performance led to the development of a research component within the department. From the mid-1960s to date, under Drs. Rehr, Rosenberg, and Blumenfield, and with the able consultation of Dr. Irwin Epstein, the social work staff has published almost 1,000 peer-reviewed articles, chapters, edited books, and books and in non–social work magazines that had an emphasis on public health education (see Chapter 8).

The marketing of social services implemented by Dr. Gary Rosenberg furthered revenue production from ambulatory care services.

The value of services was publicized to other health care professionals and to key institutional sources such as industry, further spreading the social-health concept of care. Dr. Rosenberg drew on Dr. Andrew Weissman's skills to develop the Employee Assistance Program, which made social-environmental services and consultation available to all employees and to the patients of the attending staff. The creation of public health and prevention programs emerged from the marketing perspective and from the academic association with the Department of Community and Preventive Medicine. The creation of employee wellness programs to enhance health and provide knowledge to those interested in health maintenance was piloted with Mount Sinai employees and then marketed to corporations and communities interested in wellness. Grants were obtained to increase health promotion through the creation of community programs to enhance better nutrition and exercise and reduce health hazards such as smoking and use of pesticides. While school health services were a part of Mount Sinai's services to the community, social work expanded these services by providing programs designed to enhance opportunities to children of the East Harlem community and to interest them in health and science careers. The Edith K. Ehrman Health Education Center was established to support these efforts and fostered health education for the geriatric population of East Harlem by providing direct health education services to the nine senior centers then existing in East Harlem. Each of these efforts was created and led by social work with the help of other professionals. Pregnancy prevention programs were designed to reduce the risk of those young girls who were vulnerable to early sexual experiences leading to pregnancy and childbirth. Programs were designed to support those young girls and boys who already had children to enhance their parenting skills, keep them in school, and prevent further unwanted pregnancies. Each of these programs was initially funded by the Auxiliary Board or the hospital and then funded by nonbudgetary sources.

Dr. Rosenberg was instrumental in bringing the publication *Social Work in Health Care* to Mount Sinai, becoming the editor. The publication had been founded by the late Sylvia Clarke—both Ms. Clarke as editor and the journal came to Mount Sinai's Social Work Department. Several of its staff including past and present directors are on its editorial board, as well as on the editorial board of *Health and So-*

cial Work, the NASW publication. The success of the journal allowed Drs. Rosenberg and Weissman to recommend a new publication, the *Journal of Social Work and Mental Health*, which was launched in 2002.

The Social Work Services Department of the Mount Sinai Medical Center has been a model for service, education, and research since its formal beginnings in 1906, with the assistance of a remarkable Auxiliary Board, innovative administrators, and socially oriented physicians. The department evolved, bringing in new programs for vulnerable groups, drawing on the medical center's services, and enhancing the quality of the staff's performance and institutional services. The service and study enterprises reflect the steady growth of this department as they related to societal changes and to the community demands (see Chapter 6).

Periods of fiscal difficulties required the department's staff "to do more with less." In the late 1920s, when Mrs. Fanny Mendelsohn was director of social services, she faced a problem of increased demand for services and the need for a qualified staff. Formal social work education was still in its early stages, and the need for a knowledgeable staff required a special training program. Mrs. Mendelsohn wrote of the status of the department's social workers at that time and of the need to introduce a continuing educational program to sustain quality clinical services (see Chapter 6).

Fifty years ago Doris Siegel, one year after she became director of the Department of Social Work Services, presented a paper at Massachusetts General Hospital titled "A Comprehensive Approach to Social Services in a Health Agency."* We are reprising that presentation since it cites a set of professional convictions that clearly support social work functions in serving patients and families in a health care team. In addition, she notes social work's essential roles in education, program development, community planning, and research. She also cited the "blocks" social work faced in achieving a health care professional partnership in a medical setting (see Chapter 6).

As we have come into the twenty-first century, in the cost containment practices evidenced in governmental health care policy, in pri-

---

*Doris Siegel, "A Comprehensive Approach to Social Service in a Health Agency." Presented at the Fiftieth Anniversary of the Social Service Department, Massachusetts General Hospital, Boston, MA, 1955.

vate insurance, and in managed care coverage we see the erosion of social-health care from a social utility available to those in need to a privatized commercial health care system available to those who can pay for services. The changing face of health care has resulted in an impact on its affordability, accessibility, and availability. As institutions and health care providers face major cuts in reimbursements for their services, they have been forced to implement markedly reduced services. Those that essentially deal with marginal groups with limited ability to pay for their care have been especially affected.

The social-health care model that had transposed medical care to a comprehensive diagnostic and treatment program for individuals, with a commitment to its community for their health care, is facing a compromised delivery resulting in minimalized services.

Fifty years after Doris Siegel defined the problem, have we overcome the "blocks"? Is medical care provided in the context of social-health care delivery? Does a comprehensive approach to social-health services have to be revisited? Is history repeating itself even as social change makes more demands on the health care field?

Chapter 6

Social Work's Past Shapes the Present

INTRODUCTION

The following two papers were presented by the directors of the social service department of The Mount Sinai Hospital. The first paper by Mrs. Fanny L. Mendelsohn was published in 1933 and describes her perception of the level of the social work staff and her recognition of the need to introduce staff education to better serve the hospital's patient population.

The 1920s and 1930s were times in which nurses largely staffed the few social service programs that existed in hospitals. Social services were essentially on-the-job learning experiences. The schools of social work were just coming into their own. Attitude and commitment to working with the sick had to be tested. Mrs. Mendelsohn introduced a staff educational program that reflected her vision of the need for quality practice. As one reads about the experience, one sees the sound beginnings for what has advanced into the need for continuing staff education in all social work agencies to achieve quality and accountability of services.

Fifty years ago Doris Siegel, then director of social work services of The Mount Sinai Hospital in New York City (of just one year) presented a paper at the fiftieth anniversary of Massachusetts General Hospital. She challenged her audience to consider "a comprehensive approach to social services in a health agency." In 1955 Ms. Siegel looked to the past and identified the evolving profession of "medical social work." She identified the need for standards for departments in health settings, recognizing the work of the professional associations. Most critically, she identified the essential functions, lodging them in a social service commitment, a responsibility for education of social workers and other health care professionals, and the need to study and evaluate practices through assessing accountability to the clients, the institution, and others. She noted a process had to exist in multi-professional settings that ensured collaboration with other health care providers and administrators and most important a collaboration between the social work staff and its administrator. She cited that it was a staff's awareness of their direct services, as well as their social services, that led to institutional program enhancement. She was committed to the institution's responsibility for services to its own community and for engaging local residents in making care accessible.

In 1955 Doris Siegel identified the processes and the "blocks" to be dealt with in order to offer comprehensive social services. The challenge today to the social workers in health settings and to social work educators is, "do the same issues and blocks" in their roles need to be addressed fifty years later in order to provide comprehensive care for those in need? Today, the challenge the public and health care providers face is the question, "will medical care revisit George Baehr's and Doris Siegel's concept of comprehensive social-health programs?"

AN EXPERIMENT IN STAFF EDUCATION CONDUCTED AT THE SOCIAL SERVICE DEPARTMENT OF THE MOUNT SINAI HOSPITAL: A 1932 PERSPECTIVE*

In order to understand fully the reasons which prompted The Mount Sinai Hospital Social Service Department to undertake a program of staff education, it is necessary to go back several years to the time when the growth of our department was so rapid that it became increasingly difficult to obtain properly trained personnel. It has been our policy from the very beginning to attach a social worker to a service or clinic only when the chief had made a strong personal plea for one; with the increased specialization in medicine and the steadily awakening consciousness of the medical profession to the usefulness of the social worker, one physician after the other presented his needs for our assistance.

---

*This paper was written by Fanny L. Mendelsohn, Director of Social Service Department 1923-1953, The Mount Sinai Hospital, New York City, and originally published in *Hospital Social Service,* Vol. XXVII (1), June 1933, pp. 54-58.

When I took charge of the department in 1923, the staff consisted of 26 persons. In 1929 when we felt the need for staff education most keenly, our personnel had increased to 47. The turnover on our staff was very heavy, increasing materially the need for constantly recruiting new workers.

During this period we were forced to employ workers who had little or no previous experience in hospital social work, using to an increasing degree the apprenticeship method. New appointees were obtained from four sources. From the nursing group we selected those who had had experience in the public health field and nurses who had spent three months in the Social Service Department and who had shown particular adaptability during that time. From the family case work group we took workers with no hospital background; from schools for social work, graduates, who as well as the workers from the family case work field needed supervision and tutorial work in order to carry medical case work responsibilities. Also we appointed a few individuals with secretarial experience in social service, who had good educational background and who had shown an aptitude in dealing with people and leadership within the Social Service Department.

Overtures were made to several local colleges and schools for social work to help us give our workers the particular area of social work theory needed for adequate functioning in the Hospital. None of these schools could come to our assistance at that time, and it seemed the only solution at the moment was to try out an experimental form of staff education, with no other objective than that of meeting the particular needs of our own department. We selected a person who was available for part-time work and was qualified both from the point of view of having had actual ground work experience in the field of hospital social work and who, in addition, had the qualifications necessary for a teacher.

Several years ago the Social Service Department received a gift of $50,000, the interest of which was to be used for experimental work. As our most immediate need was to work on behalf of sick children.

The newly appointed staff educator spent a month in the Children's Social Service Department and the Children's Clinic in order to familiarize herself sufficiently with the Hospital and the Social Service Department to draw up a tentative plan for staff for more adequately trained workers, it was felt that the income from this fund could not be used to better advantage than to finance a project in staff education. On October 1, 1930, she began her work on a part-time basis. It was noticed with great satisfaction from the very outset that she had the interest and wholehearted participation of the entire staff.

The original idea was to take the new appointees, but the winters of 1930 and 1931 proved unusual in that there was very little movement in personnel. Everyone, who held a position, played safe by retaining the same. The program had to be changed somewhat and certain selected members already on the staff were included.

During the first year we took three workers from the Children's Department. This proved unwise because the work there was very heavy, and in case of illness of a social worker, which occurred on several occasions, an additional burden was put on every member of that particular department. It is now our policy to take only one worker from a department and have as many different departments as possible represented. From this new method of selection we found that we had attained another objective, as for example the cardiac and asthma workers with the slow turnovers versus the gynecological and pediatric workers with rapid turnovers present different problems, giving a broader area of teaching material, thereby enlarging the students' horizon.

As the Hospital is investing considerable money by permitting the workers to participate for at least four or five hours each week over a period of eight months taken from the working schedule plus the instructor's salary, we felt justified in placing some responsibility on the workers to whom the course of eight months is offered. Therefore a letter is sent to each candidate, informing her that she is expected to remain in the department at least one year after the completion of the course, and that her salary remains stationary during this period, after which it will be reviewed. We further tell the candidates that as this form of training is of considerable expense to the Hospital, we only wish to include such workers who are keenly interested in Hospital Social Service and wish to remain in that field. We demand an answer in writing signifying willingness to comply with the above requirements. We endeavor to make it clear to the workers that the course is not offered as a substitute for professional training, but on the contrary we advise professional training if at all possible.

The plan followed has been to give an individual conference of 1-1/2 hours each week to each student selected for the experiment, as well as one conference of 1-1/2 hours per week to the whole group. At the individual conference the worker presents a current case for study, or raises points in case work application on active cases which baffle her. She may also discuss ideas she has found in her reading and which she would like to evaluate in terms of her hospital case work theory. At the same time record writing comes in for its share of attention.

At the weekly group conference a topic of current interest to the entire department, such as: planning for the care of dependent children; interviews; the best methods of achieving results through analysis of current cases being carried by members of the group, etc., are discussed.

At the beginning the same reading assignments were given to all members of the group, and the workers were requested to spend at least one evening a week in reading. However, the instructor soon found that the needs and curiosity of each worker led her into different channels of interest, so a detailed bibliography covering the whole field of case work was made available for the group with the understanding that each would direct her own reading.

During the second year the workers have two one-hour periods per month of individual conference, with suggested reading.

To report on a project which has been functioning a short time is hazardous when only ten have shared in the experiment. One worker did not keep her word and left after six months; two workers were considered unsuited for the work and were asked to resign. The other seven have greatly benefited by this service. They have developed considerably and the quality of their work has improved to a marked degree.

The following excerpt of a statement written by one of the students will give you a picture of how the staff worker feels about this opportunity.

> I have participated in three types of instructions: individual, group discussion and staff conference, each of which was under the able and interesting guidance of the staff educator.
>
> In the first, the individual conference, we discussed cases which I selected. I analyzed the problems and tried to analyze the treatment. The application of treatment, planned with my instructor, was carried out by me in the clinic with the patients and at times with various agencies. From this method of instruction,

I have developed clearer insight into the use of case work technique.

The group conference was held once a week. This group was composed of members of the staff receiving individual instruction. At these classes we had more time to think aloud in case work. While each case presented a different problem, there was a common point of view of the basic needs such as:

Financial needs or assistance
Plan for placement of children
Plan for chronic institutionalization
Adjusting the personality, etc.

The staff discussion included the entire social service staff. At this discussion group we obtained a picture of the procedure in the Hospital as a whole, and an inkling on what is being done in services other than the one with which each of us is connected.

There is a social aspect about these staff meetings. The workers are scattered in the various departments of the Hospital and only at these meetings do they all come together, and it is most enjoyable to exchange ideas and to consider together important social problems.

In conclusion, this privilege of attending the instructive groups has given me a bird's eye view of the newer methods used in social case work, which has enabled me to approach my work with keener insight and system. I am now better able to analyze the problems at hand and apply appropriate treatment more adequately.

Our weekly staff conferences have also been conducted by the staff educator, and at that time each worker has a chance to discuss an active case and present it to the whole department. Naturally, every opportunity is seized to use the different situations as teaching material.

One of the difficulties encountered in the beginning was the question of division of labor between the various administration areas within the department, the case adviser, the assistant director, who also supervises some case work, and the staff educator. We found that an occasional overlapping of function cannot be avoided. Through mutual understanding and closest cooperation, we have been able to work in greatest harmony. The staff educator is bound to come upon certain administrative problems which she discusses with me frankly, and which in several instances have helped me greatly with the direction of the department.

Another most gratifying outgrowth of this experiment is the stimulation which has been given to the whole department. The workers are following the experiment with keenest interest and a number of the more experienced workers have come to me asking for the privilege of being allowed to join the class next year.

Staff education at The Mount Sinai Hospital, although still in the experimental stage, has proved its value. We fully realize that the success of such an undertaking depends a great deal upon the instructor, and we feel that we have been very fortunate in our selection.

A COMPREHENSIVE APPROACH TO SOCIAL SERVICE IN A HEALTH AGENCY: A 1955 PERSPECTIVE*

Medical social work has made tremendous progress over the years since it began here at Massachusetts General Hospital. As the program so well illustrates, medical social workers have been accepted as an integral part of the health team in the care of the patient. As workers in the health setting our contribution is sought in many areas of teaching and planning.

We have established certain objectives and a body of content for our professional discipline. We have set down principles that form the base for our professional practice. We have blueprinted a structure and organization through which we can best operate. These facts are primary and fundamental in any consideration of a comprehensive approach to social services in a health agency.

From the beginning, medical social work has carried on many functions in the hospital and later in the health department or voluntary health association. In making our contribution in this important area of human need, health, we have used two channels: (1) direct services to patients and (2) work with others in strengthening various services.

---

*This paper was written by Doris Siegel, Director of Social Service Department, 1953-1970, The Mount Sinai Hospital, New York City.

Early in our analysis of what we do, we set down in the Statement of Standards (1949) the five functions we felt were appropriate. These were social casework, program planning, community planning, educational activities, and research. Gradually over the years, we have seen that in carrying out these functions various processes are used. These we have identified in two ways: (1) processes characteristic of social work—social casework, social group work and community organization in social work—and (2) those shared with other professions—consultation, administration, and teamwork.

Back of all these functions of the social worker is the same basic social philosophy; all necessitate the same understanding of the individual, his behavior and his social relationships. All these functions have grown out of the needs of patients and represent the part taken by social work in conjunction with medical and administrative leadership in meeting their needs. All the processes used in carrying out these functions require skill.

A Look to the Past

Although medical social workers recognized very early that the various functions were essential in any comprehensive social service program related to comprehensive medical care, in the beginning greater attention was focused on social casework as the core function, at least in the hospital. We understood much less about the other activities. We were not ready to look at interrelationships among functions, nor what the relationship was between the various processes.

Yet some thinking along these lines was evident even in these early days. In 1940, in the report of the third study of function "Some Aspects of Casework in a Medical Setting" (Bartlett, 1940), some excellent questions are posed. Although social casework was seen as the base of all concepts in social work, its applicability to other functions was recognized, and the direction for further analysis highlighted.

The expansion of medical social work into health departments, perhaps more than any other factor, pushed forward the analysis of all these responsibilities. In this new setting, social workers were asked to think and plan for more people and were required to examine what relationship could and did exist between social casework and the other functions. The Children's Bureau, Medical Social Work Section, took leadership in this effort, calling together a representative group of practitioners and teachers and coming out with a report (Baker and Siegel, 1953).

During this period and since, many new questions have been raised and some answers found. Miss Bartlett's paper for the annual meeting of the American Association of Medical Social Workers, May 1951, was both provocative and significant. Her discussion on "Some Perspectives in Public Health Social Work" (Bartlett, 1954), and on "Influence of Setting on Social Work Practice" (Bartlett, 1951), pointed out the vitality and interdependence of casework and program building. Of importance also have been the considerations of a sub-committee on administration of the Practice Committee of the American Association of Medical Social Workers. A report "Administration in Social Service in the Medical Setting" (Moss, 1952-53) raises many interesting questions on the use of the administrative process by medical social workers. Other sub-committees of both the Practice and Education Committees of the American Association of Medical Social Workers are in the process of examining other functions and processes being used in social service departments of hospitals and social work sections or units of health departments or voluntary health agencies.

Of considerable interest is the fact that a Joint Committee of the American Association of Medical Social Workers and the American Association of Psychiatric Social Workers is working on a revised "Statement of Standards to be met by Social Service Departments in Hospitals." It may be that some of the functions will be clarified and that others may emerge in this statement. Social work in relation to health and medical care has not and cannot stand still. Affected on the one hand by medicine, and on the other by social work, medical social work must be responsive to need for change and grow accordingly.

All these efforts have focused certain questions once again for us. What is the interrelationship between functions? Between processes? How can sound balance be maintained between functions and processes? As social services grow and change, what difference in balance does this suggest? What dictates priority? emphasis? What factors affect the decisions that must be made?

These problems can be relegated to the little niche reserved for "administration," mainly for the director of the social service department or the chief of the medical social work section but they shouldn't be. Such an approach is narrow and limited. The basic point of view of a department or section has a vital import for each member of the staff. The understanding based on thinking through and resolution of questions of relationships, and the interdependence of various functions and of processes affect practice and in this way affect each practitioner. Also in a smaller way each worker must face these same questions in regard to his or her area of medical services or areas of responsibility.

In spite of excellent beginnings, our knowledge at this point is too slim to permit a blueprint. We need to do more thinking. We need to do a better job of sifting our experience for those leavens of future accomplishments. At this time, we can look at practice and perhaps outline some principles and suggestions that may serve as catalysts.

A Look at the Present

The pattern followed by most social service departments in the past, and today, is first to develop the social casework function; then to move into educational activities; and finally to enter into program planning, community planning and research. In the health agency, this was the pattern also but with more emphasis on working with others through consultation and teamwork.

For a time an effort was made to meet all needs through consultation. But gradually, many workers in health departments have come to feel that direct help—casework—must find a place somewhere in a program but in collaboration with other health care providers.

In most hospitals today, social casework continues to be the core function. Where our demonstration has been skillful, it is the service for which we are constantly requested. Our setting, the hospital, is one in which change takes place constantly. New interns, new residents, new nurses (not to mention new social workers!) come and go. Social casework constantly needs interpretation, not through words alone, but through demonstration—and this need is always with us. We have, however, established our individualized service of social casework firmly and soundly as a valuable and valued service.

In the health department setting, the place of social casework is more controversial. Some workers believe other professional people can be helped to consider the social component in an individual situation within their competence and that it is unrealistic to expect the medical social worker to provide direct casework service to the individual. I believe that this service must be available somewhere in the program. The individual patient and his needs must be the base for our knowledge, security, and learning. The worker cannot carry on effectively with other responsibilities completely separated from social casework.

The process of consultation is today much more developed in the health department or (health) associations than it is in the hospital. Community organization is used in a limited way in both settings. All directors of departments or units do carry out the administrative process in attempting to integrate various parts of the program. Any picture of practice today would certainly show the process of teamwork although much of it not sufficiently utilized in many instances. Participation by the social worker in program development, using whatever processes are needed, is being carried on to some extent in the hospital, but to a much greater extent in the health department and voluntary health association.

Practice, of course, depends upon the stage of development of social service in any agency. Those agencies where social service is just beginning are at a different stage in practice than those where it has been in existence many years. I am sure that Massachusetts General Hospital faces somewhat different problems than other hospitals and that its practice reflects its many years of established sound experience. Departments newly developed or even reorganized have to repeat some of the growing pains of previous ventures even though they certainly begin much ahead and move forward much faster.

The Setting in Which We Work

As a background for our discussion, we will look briefly at the setting of the health agency. Medical social work developed its functions out of the needs presented by patients in this setting. So too, must the setting influence interrelationships between functions and any decisions and judgments on balance between them.

In the hospital or health department, social work cannot exist in an ivory tower. We are surrounded by people, many of them with social and emotional needs closely related to their medical needs. Our presence in the midst of the setting, close to the reality of the needs of people cannot help but affect our selection and intake. This is both an asset and a problem. On the one hand, we have a wonderful opportunity to find people who can use our help. On the other hand, we become full of anxiety and almost overwhelmed by the great need that exists. I believe the opportunity this presents is greater than the problem it creates, however.

In the hospital or health department the social worker faces certain difficulties in that he or she must relate to both the administrative and the clinical aspects of the program. One is always dealing with these two strands—and sometimes these strands pull the worker in different directions. They may prevent achieving balance between functions.

The hospital or health department, as has been so well pointed out by Simmons and Wolff (1954), presents a sociological entity. It sets certain patterns and expectations. Everyone must fit into this framework—the patient as well as the staff. This has a bearing on our discussion.

Functions and Processes: Their Relationship

We have clearly demonstrated the interdependence of the various responsibilities of the social worker in the health agency. As stated in the monograph "Medical Social Services for Children," "one . . . (function) grows from and is strengthened by the other. One flows naturally into the other" (Baker and Siegel, 1953).

It is, of course, possible to develop one phase of service to the exclusion of others. Superficially this may seem to focus effort on one responsibility and consequently strengthen it; but, in the long run, such an effort may weaken the service, may result in its becoming unrelated, limited, sterile. Developing various functions slowly and at a favorable time may in the final analysis strengthen all functions.

The relationship between social casework and teaching is obvious. Casework, dealing as it does with living people, the problems they face, and the ways we use in helping them, gives the worker the security to teach. Other professions similarly keep their confidence in us if we continue to draw our knowledge from actual work with people. Material drawn from our patients makes the difference between theoretical, intellectual teaching and teaching that reaches into emotional meaning. In turn, our participation in teaching reflects back into our casework. The questions and issues raised by students pose problems requiring analysis and stimulate us to explore and push our ideas further.

Both of these functions contribute heavily to the social worker's participation in program planning within the health agency. Out of that experience with people, the social worker speaks forcefully on the need for certain policies and procedures. As the worker tries to help people through social casework, he/she recognizes gaps in the program of services and works for the initiation and development of ways to close them. Social casework helps one identify these areas and gives conviction to what is said. Naturally, one may need to add a number of one's experiences and impressions together. Or he/she may need to move into research for special study and for accumulation of data. Results of such study or research may be used in program development, in standard setting and even in service to people, directly or through consultation to others.

All of these functions as they move back and forth certainly may lead to participation in community planning. Often it is a step, and a short one at that, from using material from casework, research, teaching to influencing program within the health agency and with the community. How well the social worker in the health agency can speak on the need for foster homes for handicapped children! How vividly then social work can point to the value of specially planned housing for the sick aged in preserving the mental health of this ever increasing group in our community! How strongly we can speak on the meaning of preventive services if our young people are to achieve their potentialities!

The worker uses all the processes on the job. Certain functions require the use of more than one process. For example, in participating in planning service, workers offer consultation to the program or hospital director, use group work skills in working with committees, and exercise teamwork along with other professional personnel. A worker may give casework service to a family and terminate one's own responsibility. But as a new problem arises, without renewing the contact with the family, the worker may be asked to give consultation to another professional member of the health team on certain psychosocial factors operating in the situation.

Functions may be carried out with vision and imagination or in a truly myopic fashion. To do the latter means overlooking the possibilities and opportunities open to us to make a meaningful contribution on a wider basis. Judgment on timing, priority, emphasis must always operate, however. A basic philosophy is imperative and must underlie whatever procedure or plan we follow. A philosophy which stresses a broad approach and an alertness to opportunities for wider contribution would seem to have strength for us.

Balancing Functions

If we accept the basic premise of the desirability of a social service department or unit within a health agency carrying a number of functions and using a number of processes, how can balance be achieved? What, for that matter, is balance in this context? Does it mean an equal proportion of time and emphasis on all functions? Does this proportion change in moving from the beginning of a department to a well-established department? What factors make for change during this process?

Balance must, of course, be relative. We certainly cannot allot so much time or so much emphasis to any one function. A definite and exact time schedule even with medical and administrative help could not be expected from a worker. Certain general ideas have grown out of experience that may be helpful in achieving a measure of balance in social services. These in turn may help us define certain principles we can use.

Balance cannot be achieved unless the various functions that go into making up the whole—and the whole itself—are recognized. This implies a process of planning and decision-making. It means decisions consciously arrived at, rather than "slid into." It means defining and setting down goals; and then reviewing and evaluating them to see how far we have come, what changes in direction are necessary, what new objectives need to be set.

Although a quantitative description of functions is not possible nor desirable, any social service department or unit within a health agency should carry the generally accepted functions described in the "Statement of Standards" and in "Medical Social Service for Children." Responsibility for other activities may be carried also but this should be minimal. Otherwise, the weight would not seem to be on those activities which are central and basic to social work and which permit the worker to make an appropriate social work contribution directly or indirectly to patient care and hospital or health agency service.

If the major part of the social worker's effort is directed toward administrative management in the hospital or health department, then he/she is not doing a social work job, even though one may be using social work knowledge and skill. A job is a social work job when

(a) the primary purpose is a social work purpose
(b) the job requires the use of a range of social work knowledge and skill in one of their recognized manifestations; e.g., casework, etc.
(c) the job is professional social work clearly enough to be distinguished as such by patients and other professional people

Although one particular function may receive special and concentrated attention, other functions must also be developed eventually. This means conviction on our part that all the functions are valid and a need for alertness to opportunities to move from one to another. We may, of course, have to delay actual steps to use the opportunities present; and, in a small set-up, this may mean reducing certain functions to occasional and informal efforts.

Balance cannot be reached overnight. In relation to certain functions, some safeguards are necessary. *The teaching of our own profession or of other professions should be undertaken only if the practice of social casework has developed soundly in the hospital, and casework plus consultation is available in the health department program.* As was well stated in "Widening Horizons in Medical Education" (Commonwealth Fund of New York, 1948), teaching should be based on well-founded practice and the student should be able to see demonstration of our service. Otherwise, our teaching is not sound, and inevitably results in confusion. To establish little islands for students in hospitals and other health agencies, as some schools of social work do, seems to be unreal and artificial. Here I would rather see focusing on one function, casework, primarily and working toward including other functions.

An emphasis on research cannot be substituted for a good program of practice. Certainly, small study endeavors are part of the way to keep practice vital, but *we should not attempt an all-out effort on research before practice is well established and firm.* I would question also participation in medical research without provision of service. This, of course, may be dependent upon the medical plan. It may not be desirable to have the same person who is doing the research also give the casework service, but its availability in a program must be assured.

Balance cannot be achieved in a vacuum. *A sufficient number of staff—qualified and able—must be available for social service of high quality to be given and for the various functions to be carried out.* It is unrealistic to talk in terms of a balanced grouping of functions, wherein we move from one to the other, unless enough staff are provided to make this possible.

The amount of emphasis given to any one function even within a reasonably well staffed department still needs examination. We know that the essential nature of social casework limits the number of individuals to whom a social worker can given a good quality of service. This principle applied equally to the social worker's ability to give a good quality of service in relation to teaching, program planning, community planning, etc. With the many demands on us it is easy to succumb to the "doing something on everything" disease. On the other hand, we cannot ignore all but one part of one function. The recognition we achieve in medical school teaching, and its importance, can make us forget our possible contribution in nursing education. We may enjoy community planning to the point of serving the health agency almost secondarily. We need to guard against spreading ourselves too thin in any area though still aware of the whole. Again the balance we seek to achieve is delicate and fine.

Blocks to Balance

What are some of the problems interfering with achieving of balance among functions and, perhaps even before that, to taking on various functions?

Some of the blocks exist within the worker himself. It is true, and we have all tested this in our own experience, that the worker just out of school has all he can do to begin cementing with practice what was learned in social casework. He/she is not ready nor does one have the skill to take on and to use any other function to any extent, nor to use a process other than casework. All too often the worker does not recognize that another function might be desirable or that it even exists.

The beginning worker cannot be expected to have the skill. But he/she can be expected, however, to have a positive attitude.

Yet many times this positive attitude is not present. Although in training an increasing effort is being made to reach our students in this way and to help them recognize implications for program planning, community planning, research, much of it is not getting results and more and renewed efforts are required. Sometimes teachers in our schools, and often, our field work instructors, do not have a conviction that transmits itself to students. The wide open, tremendous field of casework practice always seems to hold more promise and excitement for most of us. If, however, we can help students and workers see the implications of case situations for other functions and the way these functions can relate to the case situation, we shall be bringing other ways into the process of helping our patients.

Another block disturbing balance lies in our social service hierarchy. Too often as directors of departments or units we clutch certain functions to ourselves. We do this from mixed motives. Sometimes in an effort to protect our staff we seal them off from administrative controls above us and carry the burden of interpretations, and the responsibility to use this chance to influence policy if it is present. Sometimes we may feel we can handle problems requiring administrative action with more dispatch and do not trouble to make the kind of preparation or arrange for post discussion that is necessary if our worker accompanies us. Granted no one way to do this exists, nevertheless we might well make more of an effort to give our workers a living experience in participating in program planning. After all, our social work education is based on learning through directed experience.

This same point may be made in regard to participation in community planning. We are increasingly recognizing that there is tremendous value in representation by administrative and other hospital personnel in various community activities—committees, conferences, etc. Perhaps this principle can apply equally to members of the social service department staff other than the director. *All too often this kind of representation is limited to him and not shared widely.* Hospitals might well follow the example of health departments or voluntary health agencies in this respect.

Wider participation cannot be automatically assumed. Workers should be more experienced and secure in their representation. Where this can be planned the total department or unit benefits as well as do the various responsibilities carried.

The readiness of the health agency to accept various functions, and perhaps the function of the agency itself, is of course, a most significant factor in achieving balance. Health departments are much more accustomed than hospitals to program development and to using the contribution of all professional personnel in the process. They have found that it works. A more extensive and intensive use of the social worker in program development would be expected. Also, the health department is clearer about its responsibility to the community and about its concern for many people. Although many hospitals are strong forces in community planning, and more should be, the health department is more engaged in this, and naturally the social worker is more involved in community planning and consultation. The hospital in turn with its focus on care of the patient, teaching and research, uses the social worker more in these functions. The health department has always used consultation more than the hospital but hospitals are now putting emphasis on this important process. In all instances we need to work to interpret the importance of the other functions and to attempt to increase readiness of the agency to use social workers in performing them. Balance can certainly come about in this way.

Criteria for Balance

The underlying factor in achieving balance among functions is of course, judgment—judgment in assessing a situation, in setting goals, in determining ways to reach goals and in planning timing. Each worker brings their training and experience to any judgment that needs to be made. We have, however, learned certain principles which can affect our judgment.

Short-term goals must be weighed against long term objectives. What may seem to advance social service on a short time basis, because it increases prestige, gives recognition, etc., may in the long run deter the social service department or unit from making its best contribution to the care of people.

As we respect our own contribution, as we are secure in what we have to give in each and every function, we are better able to communicate this effectively and demonstrate it concretely to others. Security brings with it flexibility and an ability to change if this seems desirable.

We need to bring our basic understanding of people and motivation into our effort to develop balance among functions. Listening and knowing what people are really saying, building on strength and disciplining ourselves are essential in improving our judgment and acting on it.

Both new and ongoing activities should be tested for their appropriateness and effect on other activities. Constant evaluation is the touchstone to growth.

No magic formula exists to help us on timing. But knowing our situation and the individuals involved helps. So do patience and ability to withstand external and internal pressures. Courage often is an important ingredient. Sometimes we must work on "just plain instinct," and hope for the best.

Issues

Although some ideas on balance between functions have been reaffirmed and some have emerged, a number of issues still remain. No danger exists in social work that answers will outstrip questions.

We need to look further at what I have called "other activities" which are being assumed by the social worker in a health agency. I do not consider these as professional and believe they, in fact, detract from our professional contribution even though some of our compatriots are of the opinion that some of these activities—follow-up, handling of appliances, referral to visiting nurse service—have social implications. In some health agencies, these activities are being handled routinely by case aides and referred selectively to social service when needed. Is this a semi-professional or a clerical function? Should the case aide be a member of the social service department staff or part of administration? We need to define what is professional in our service, and what semi-professional activities are carried by our departments. It may be that contrary to the practice of the social agency which carries some semi-professional tasks, these may be delegated to others in the health agency.

The whole question of the meaning of working with clinical and administrative personnel needs to be explored further. How we balance pulls in two directions requires more discussion. We share this conflict with others in the health agency and joint discussion may be in order.

Further consideration needs to be given to the one-man social service department or unit. What special adaptations does the lone worker make in achieving balance? For even in this instance balance must still remain the goal.

In this paper we have spoken of consultation as a *process*. We are not clear as yet whether it will prove to be a *function*. Other professions may have arrived at greater clarity. We have also mentioned the use of group work skills by the social caseworker. Actually, we need to examine much more closely whether and when the caseworker can use such skills. Ideally, every student worker in a school of social work would have had some exposure to social group work in field and class teaching. We know this has not been achieved. Yet today much discussion and activity by the caseworker is going on and is variously called "group counseling," "group therapy," etc. Where casework and group work are interrelated needs much more discussion. In considering processes, we need also to examine whether those processes carried by all professions take on special social work characteristics when adapted by the social worker.

Final balance is never achieved and should not be. The center for balance generally remains the same, but social services in any health agency must always be responsive to growth and change within the agency and within the community. Changes in the balance among functions should reflect such external change. As some health agencies offer more help to private physicians, we should be able to add consultation on social and emotional problems in patients. This may mean a shift in the balance among functions. As long as we see the long-range goals, recognize the problems, and yet meet the demands of the situation as flexibly and creatively as possible, a balance will be maintained.

This entire paper is based on the assumption that social work has a contribution to make to the health agency and that this contribution is made through carrying a number of functions and using a number of processes. Social work shares with all members of the health team the basic objective of helping people meet the social and emotional problems blocking their positive health, and creating a climate in which adjustment and health can flourish. Together, all the health professions can work toward doing a better job in one area of human need—health.

REFERENCES

American Association of Medical Social Workers, "A Statement of Standards to be Met by Medical Social Service Departments in Hospital and Clinics," Washington, DC, 1949, Revised, 8 pp.

Baker, E. M., and Siegel, D. "Medical Social Services for Children," Children's Bureau Publication 343, Washington, DC, 1953, 49 pp.

Bartlett, H. M. "Influence of Setting on Social Work Practice." Proceedings of Institute on Social Work Practice in the Medical and Psychiatric Setting, University of Pittsburgh, June 1951, pp. 11-26 mimeographed.

Bartlett, H. M. "Medical Social Work Today and Tomorrow," *Medical Social Work,* Vol. 1 (1), September 1951, pp. 1-18.

Bartlett, H. M. "Some Aspects of Social Casework in a Medical Setting," George Banta Publishing Co., 1940, 270 pp.

Bartlett, H. M. "Some Perspectives in Public Health Social Work," *Children,* Vol. 1 (1), January-February 1954, pp. 21-25.

Joint Committee of the Association of American Medical Colleges and American Association of Medical Social Workers, "Widening Horizon in Medical Education," Commonwealth Fund of New York, 1948, 228 pp.

Moss, C. "Administration in Social Service in the Medical Setting," 1952-1953.

Selected Papers and Reports, Fiftieth Anniversary Celebration, Social Service Department, Massachusetts General Hospital, Boston, MA, 1955, pp. 104-118.

Simmons, L. W., and Wolff, H. G. "Social Science in Medicine," Russell Sage Foundation, New York, NY, 1954, 254 pp.

Chapter 7

Social Work Research in Health Care: Studies That Affect Practice

> The bottom line in research utilization in social work is that research findings must have utility for practice. Elegance of design, sophistication of statistics and the soundness of theory, are all beside the point if the problem that is addressed has little relevance to client needs or service delivery. (Jenkins, 1990, p. 3)

It is to these two objectives that social work study of its services, irrespective of delivery location, that this chapter addresses: (1) to enhance the clinical practice relevant to clients and their needs and (2) to review and enhance agency service programs.

Both objectives require, no matter the means by which a study is conducted, that the findings are, in the final analysis, returned to the social work clinicians for their translation into practice and program change and to those who created programs to meet needs. This premise can certainly be argued at the micro level where learned information is to be utilized by practitioners on behalf of the clients' benefit. At the macro level, the social work profession seeks to utilize the findings of "community"-based studies on behalf of given population needs within coalitions for social action regarding policy and programmatic goals.

From 1915 (when Flexner asserted there was no evidence that social work was a profession) to the present, reference to social work research is that it should be scientifically based. While not eschewing theoretically based research, our approach has remained consistent that, in the study of an agency's social services, it should have "utility for practice"—applied social work research.

> Nearly every debate about social work's status as a profession has concentrated upon the extent to which it possess a signifi-

cant body of knowledge that is derived from scientific research, amenable to widespread discrimination (policy and program), and applicable by practitioners in ways that are both effectual and efficient (practice). (Feldman, 1992, p. xviii)

While a body of knowledge is critical, one needs to determine how it is used; this is ultimately important for those who serve in the field. The key questions that the field has had to face are: "How effective is social work and how can it become more effective?"

This chapter addresses the questions from the perspective of the utilization of studies to affect the practice and programs of social workers in a large academic medical center.

PREMISE

Social work has attempted to underpin its mission and raison d'être with scientific inquiry from its formal beginnings in the United States at the end of the nineteenth century. What is known to date about social work research is that the findings of studies of practice and its outcome "are of variable quality, making generalizations hard to draw" (Kirk, 1999, p. 306). Also, research of social work practice is complicated by multiple factors; a mosaic of inputs is involved, some of which are the "vast array of problems social workers treat, the diversity of populations served, the many social-environments from which people come, and the variety of settings (units) in which they work, et al" (Kirk, 1999, p. 309).

The question so often posed is whether social work practice is subject to scientific study. Given the complex and complicated health care concerns presented by people, it is clear that in the vast array of treatments for given disorders, no single health care discipline can claim that a known process results in a given outcome. In medical settings, inter- and multidisciplinary teams have talked about the need to develop collaborative models to understand outcomes of social-health care delivery (Dana, 1983). However, collaborative assessment still remains to be achieved. Each discipline has moved to claim its own approach of process to outcome. While this evaluation method has led to knowledge building, it has also led to more specialization and fragmentation.

Social work services in health care settings followed the pattern for self-examination of its services similar to that undertaken by its health care colleagues. However, social workers' studies held that any examination of its services had to be useful to improving care for its consumers (Jenkins, 1990).

When an institution is invested in a service delivery program, it needs to find the means to learn who it is serving, what is being given and their outcomes, along with the cost-effectiveness of those services delivered to its clientele. Some of the questions posed: Have clients been helped with their social-health problems? Are the outcomes valid? Are the clients satisfied with the results? Do the clients and clinicians agree the services have been helpful? What requires change?

For an administrator in a health care setting, the demand for accountability of the social work services comes from multiple sources, internal and external, to regulators and payers who represent their constituencies. Anecdotal case illustrations of the client's social-health situation, while valuable and descriptive in demonstrating the range of services to clients, to other health care professionals no longer justify budgetary allocations for service. It is essential to find the data that serve to inform and to evaluate the practice of the staff and the programs available to the institution's clientele.

BACKGROUND

In medical settings, a means to achieve the quality assessment of medical care has a mid-nineteenth century historical base in the United States. Florence Nightingale in the 1860s was concerned with the quality of care given on the battlefields during the Civil War—in particular the nursing care of casualties. Flexner (1915), shortly after the turn of the century, cited the deficiencies of medical education and the resultant poor medical care. Codman in 1915 following Flexner studied the care received by patients in American hospitals. His means of measurement was the "end result" of care given. His findings led the American College of Surgeons to set standards in 1918 for surgical procedures (End Stage Renal Disease Program Guidelines, 1977). The reviews of hospital services that followed were undertaken by in-house committees studying the "end result" of their own specialties. In 1951, the Joint Commission on Hospital Accreditation (currently the JCAHO) was formed by the major professional health care organizations to serve as an accreditation body of hospitals on the quality and quantity of services to patients that were offered by the institution and its professional health care staffs.

For years, services were audited by these internal peer review committees. The Social Security Act via Title 18 and 19 mandated review of professional services. Federal law in 1972 called for the establishment of professional review committees (PROs) requiring the professional accountability of a "quality assurance" (QA) of medical and institutional care. As economic difficulties were evident, affecting the reimbursement to hospitals for their services, the federal government linked quality assurance and cost containment. The federal mandate covered utilization reviews, which set standards for admission and length of stay, and discharge reviews to prevent overstays.

Diagnosis-related groups (DRGs) were introduced to set a hospitalization period for disease-specific procedures and treatment. The mandate moved hospitals to attempt to curb the ever-growing costs of inpatient stays. The requirements meant data collection was mandatory. Prior to the mandate, hospitals tended to maintain limited information about whom they admitted, and for what, except for given units of service that sought to audit their own endeavors.

Information that was collected by institutions was seen as the "private purview" of its reviewer. The information of primary interest to institutions was data needed for reimbursement, e.g., inpatient stays, outpatient visits, laboratory and other procedures—essentially for billing and personnel processing. However, by the 1980s mandated expectations included demographics, admission and discharge dates, diagnoses, and prescribed services delivered. These led to the components in disease-based inpatient lengths of stay—the DRGs.

As the technology was developed to encompass the "who," "what," "when," and "how" of medical care that the mandate called for, the outcome (what happened) remained elusive. The need to review quality of care of health care professionals and the institutions for services delivered to their patients had come under active investigation by a number of social scientists. One, in particular, Avedis Donabedian (1973), projected that quality assurance could be measured in the context of "structure, process and outcomes." The expectations of this framework required reviewing mechanisms of

- professionally developed norms, criteria, and standards;
- a data retrieval system on patients, providers, and institutions;
- a utilization review system and periodic medical care evaluation studies;
- a peer review system based on established criteria;
- a means to correct identified deficiencies related to individual and organizational performance;
- continuing education as a corrective measure; and
- a uniform information and data system for regional and cross-institutional assessments (PSRO Program Manual, 1974, p. 1).

The mandate also set the beginnings of a national data collection body via the establishment of the Uniform Hospital Discharge Data System (UHDDS) (Rehr, 1979, p. 18).

> The Joint Commission on Accreditation of Hospital Organizations (JCAHO) assigned as the formal reviewing body of hospital care, interpreted q.a. within the reviewing expectations, setting its assessment on "what" had been given to "whom." Over time the "what" appeared to be a static review which seemed not to lead to change. Q.A. was then revised to achieve essential change by mandating continuous quality improvement (c.q.i.). Present day assessments are expected to achieve change. While many assessments by institutions are taken post-delivery of service from medical chart documentation, some academic medical institutions have undertaken assessments of care concurrent with delivery (while the patient was hospitalized). The JCAHO measurement is in c.q.i.

The context implied with JCAHO's system for evaluating care is that continuous quality improvement (CQI) is lodged in the belief that the many variables reviewed—the quality of the facilities, equipment, staffing, qualifications and experience of personnel, organizational arrangements, information system, and financing—are structural standards. The assumption has been that a good structure would inevitably lead to a good process, hence a good outcome. However, there is no tested relationship that confirms good structure leads to good outcomes. Structural standards do affirm institutional quality. However, to validate outcome, the route to its study is complex and lined with multiple variables (Rehr et al., 1998, p. 66). Nevertheless, social workers with the support of the hospital's Auxiliary Board undertook to study its clinical practices and its programs. The Auxiliary Board endorsed the Department's early studies by advancing the funds to initiate them.

SOCIAL WORK STUDIES ITSELF

The social services from their beginnings had a number of means to arrive at findings based on collective review of situations. Jane Addams, Mary Richmond, Bertha Reynolds, and their colleagues and successors have looked to assess social-health problems in the community and the needs of given populations. Their joint efforts with physicians and social activists were responsible for many social-environmental and health changes.

Many of these studies (surveys) dealt with the disease impact on individuals and their families in their communities, as well as on social-health concerns. Within hospitals, the early focus of studies done jointly by doctors and social workers was to isolate the group with a common disorder to understand its impact on the quality of life. One that was prevalent in the fifties was poliomyelitis, which was epidemic after World War II and which was studied (Sweet and White, 1961). Also the pregnancies of unmarried women, particularly of teenagers, were a societal concern at that time (Young, 1950). This population was under frequent review to understand their behavior and to offer preventive care (Rehr et al., 1962, 1963).

The intent of CQI was to achieve a continuous reviewing means of those invested in service delivery. While review mechanisms were noted, major concerns surfaced:

- the "how" to define the complexities of care;
- the impact of physical, psychological, or social functioning factors;
- "who" delivers care, e.g., a doctor, a team of health care professionals, specialists;
- the procedures and treatment modalities, i.e., the instrumentalities of care;
- who are the recipients of service: the patient, the family, others, a population;

- the nature of the review, whether a caseload, a unit of service, a population;
- the external factors impacting the client system;
- and, finally, *what* is the outcome of care compliance, the optimization of quality of life?

The social workers in the health care field wanted to learn how to judge the effectiveness of social service. They needed to know what was achieved and what was not and if possible to gauge the processes that made for results. There has been much work in developing instruments to measure "goal" attainment: single-subject assessments, experimental designs, descriptive studies, process studies identifying interventive typologies, goal attainment scales, and a host of other evaluative methodologies (Berkman and Weissman, 1983).

Given the mandate to hospitals and health care practitioners to seek CQI, the social work departments, in the large academic medical centers, along with the social work section (SSWHC of the JCAHO) moved early to engage in quality review of its social services. Across the country a number of studies surfaced to capture the clientele served and their needs. What became paramount for social work in health care was the need to demonstrate the significance of social-health principles in place of what had been "essentially a biomedical model of health care delivery" and to develop a framework for quality assurance that values the social work contribution to patient-family health care.

The helping process with individuals is difficult to both define and measure. Social work is not a basic science that can produce a theoretical knowledge, even though long sought. It was nevertheless essential to solidify social work's place in multidisciplinary social-health care. Recognizing there is no theory that objectified problem-to-process-to-outcome (Donabedian, 1973) and that practice "is an art" (Schon, 1983) (not unlike the "art of medicine"), social work attempted to identify the components in its practice and in its programs.

In order to integrate social-health principles, social work leaders at The Mount Sinai Hospital believed the challenge rested with an administration-staff partnership regarding what data needed to be gathered to enhance the clinical care of patients and the department's programs. To secure the social workers' investment, they were asked to do "one-page studies" as a means to capture the social-health problems they were encountering. The approach offered a simple way to look at "presenting" problems and a few variables in their patient-family care. The objective of the one-page studies was to demonstrate the value of reflection over a time period on multiple cases in the social worker's caseload. It was expected that such periodic reviews would raise questions about one's practice or programs and subject them to change. It was also hoped that the review of cases would demystify research for practitioners and help them to recognize their contribution to self-evaluation of their services and the need for change (Rehr, 1979).

The studies undertaken at this institution and at other social work centers across the country supported the integration of a social-health focus to medical care, and at the same time they assumed a responsibility for QA, followed by CQI as mandated by the federal government and the JCAHO (Rehr, 1979; Morrison et al., 1982).

In 1967, Berkman and Rehr demonstrated in their studies of elderly inpatients their need for social service interventions. The earlier belief was that only low-income patients were social work clients. Their study determined that a biopsychosocial need was unrelated to the income level of patients. The findings of the study also documented the rationale for increased services to the private patients of the institution. The study translated patient need into a frame of reference of "problems presented" by the client system. For the hospital elderly population, it was possible to create a problem classification system (Berkman and Rehr, 1972).

The problem classification system developed at Mount Sinai was a variation on the Bellevue Hospital study of inpatients by Mary Jarrett (1946). Jarrett, based on experience, undertook a study that arrived at a formula for case-finding, i.e., those in need of social services, which she found distributed along a ratio of high/medium and low of 1/3, 1/3, and 1/3. For many years, this had been a formula (roughly adopted) by which most staffs did case-findings on their service units. However, by 1967, Rehr and Berkman translated problem classification into a screening procedure for early identification of patients and their families facing social and emotional risk related to the illness. Developing indicators of social risk screening moved social work from dependence on referrals from other health care professionals and community social agencies to autonomy of its own case-finding system (Rehr, 1982).

Social work further developed its autonomous case-finding system by examining the projected after-hospital care needs of patients in a preadmission screening procedure. By contact of to-be-admitted patients for elective medical care, trained social workers and medical students were able to advise patients and to assign social workers for social service intervention to work on the identified need (Reardon et al., 1988). The preadmission and in-hospital screening of patients became a standardized social work case-finding procedure in institutions across the country. Apart from its benefit of early and direct services to those in need, early intervention programs proved to be cost effective discharge planning. Social work contributed to cost containment by reducing length of stay, planning early for patients' post-hospital discharge needs, and ensuring that discharge plans are fulfilled by a telephone follow-up program (Simon et al., 1995).

Always, the need to learn the outcomes of social work intervention loomed large. What was the best way to dissect the complex factors in determining what is (are) responsible for "what happened" in known situations? Social work had safely achieved one aspect of "access" to care for persons with illness by its means of case-finding. It faced two major factors—what were the interventions in relation to problems identified and to what happened? Was the outcome related to the interventions? One returns always, when viewing the social and behavioral sciences, to the recognition that for the complexities of multiple variables in the human entity and environment, and to the variables in the service system, there is no unilinear cause (process) and effect that can be allocated to social work interventions. Yet, the demand for the validation and justification for a social-health model of care faced the health care professions.

After reviewing the literature (e.g., Donabedian, 1973; Starfield, 1974; Greene, 1976), we turned to the concept of "satisfaction" with services delivered as one "outcome" measure. We speculated that the voices of the consumers could lend credence to their assessment of their health care experiences to administrators, to health care providers, to regulators and reviewers, and to the social work staff itself. There was documented evidence of the consumers' responses to social service (Overton, 1960; Maluccio, 1979; Perlman, 1975).

Satisfaction as a measure of outcome has not been favored by the social science and social work researchers. Its reliability is considered too soft a variable and thus questionable. Nevertheless, the department moved ahead to look at process by having the social work staff recognize problems they identified with the client and to conceptualize a contract between client and practitioner that was mutually agreed to and would be the focus of their transaction. Drawing on the Berkman-Rehr Problem Classification as an across-the-board measure attempting to structure a problem-to-contract approach, on Reid and Epstein (1972) for task-oriented services, and on Maluccio and Marlow (1974, p. 91) for contracting, "it was possible to arrive at the formulation of a contracted mutual agreement between the client system and the worker regarding the problem to be dealt with." A series of typologies dealing with interventions or process have been forthcoming (Chernesky and Lurie, 1976; Reid, 1980). Their variations reflect the art of practice as noted by Schon in his reflections on the limitations of any defined modalities that can correlate with contractual agreements.

If one approaches the client system with the questions "Were the social work services provided helpful to you? and in what way?" one moves to obtain the opinion of those served. It is the "voice of the consumer" from which social work learns to evaluate its services.

Early on, the federal mandate to assess the quality of service led the Social Work Department to undertake a survey of consumers' opinions of the hospital care. The past methods of a mailed questionnaire to discharged patients averaged a disappointing 10 percent response rate, and findings were ineffectual for change. In conjunction with senior hospital management, social work researchers identified the areas of service and location of patients and set a four-level rating system for opinions. The survey method was via telephone to discharged patients by a trained staff. The findings were processed and shared with appropriate staff to introduce essential change. The intent was not to identify individual staff performance, but rather the quality of the services on the unit and thus practice. The Medical Center continues the use of this CQI survey (modified to today's needs) to tap patients' opinions of care, to inform staff, to introduce essential change, and to meet accreditation expectations (Morrison et al., 1982).

The concept of client satisfaction, while soft in contrast to the scientific assessment of service, does serve some functional and useful purposes. Maluccio (1979) in addressing the value for social work noted that "obtaining the views and insights of those we help is an essential means of critically examining our practice and refining our skills" (p. xii). In seeking client satisfaction with services offered and received, social work in health care has looked to three different participants in the process: the client and/or his or her proxy and the social worker. In studies undertaken by social workers, the responses show a relatively high correlation between patient and proxy respondents as to satisfaction (Rehr, 1989). Differences in responses may be related to when the survey was done, the perception of discharge planning, and the individual's perception of his health status (Showers et al., 1995). When social workers are asked for their opinion of the benefit of the social work intervention, they tend to see less benefit than their clients (Rehr, 1989). Client satisfaction studies are not without their complications. Issues as to when they are done in relation to care received, what is being asked, the personal behavior of respondents, and their health status are all factors that limit the validity of responses. On the other hand, there are benefits from patient/proxy/social worker follow-up of services given. At this medical institution, where consumer satisfaction with medical/hospital/nursing and social work services is routinely studied with a random selection of discharged patients, administration has uncovered impediments in service, program problems, limited health care instructions, and the need to deal with staff behaviors and suggestions to modify and enhance service delivery. Mechanisms to deal with change are utilized. For the institution, satisfaction findings have the potential to advance market strategies in improving care. For the health care professionals, social workers in particular, they offer a view (even if limited) to the clients' perception of social services and an opportunity to engage in both performance and program analyses. In this context, the authors mention T. Franklin Williams' claim that "research and care require each other; they interact with each other" (1988, p. 579). Consumer satisfaction studies remain one way to view the social-health enterprise from the perception of those involved in it (Ware et al., 1978).

The process of systematically viewing social-health care delivery and its benefits to clients has confronted the social scientists. The complexities are many, the interceding variables are multiple, attitudes and behaviors of recipients and practitioners are numerous, and a host of other factors do not make research neat. We have noted elsewhere "the difficulty of demonstrating a definitive causal relationship between problems-to-process-to-outcome" (Rehr et al., 1998, p. 66). Social work services like those of medicine are difficult to measure.

The other complication is who researches what. Not infrequently when social researchers are brought into institutions, they tend to alienate or avoid the clinicians, who are the usual source of information. Clinicians are not usually included in interpreting the study findings. They believe the "art of practice" has generally been ignored; and, thus, application is usually not addressed.

This social work department, wanting to be informed early and periodically, has invested in "quick and dirty" reviews, which offer an administrator a view of service delivery. Such quickies are another way of becoming informed. It has, however, in the main, for social work practice and programs enlightenment, turned to practice-based studies involving a staff-administrative partnership, with research consultation by the social worker-"researcher." Home-based social researchers on the premises who are themselves practice-focused, knowledgeable of the setting, respectful of clinician insights, and supportive of Schon's conception of "reflection-in-action," can gain the trust of practitioners and of those with whom they work (Blumenfield and Epstein, 2002).

The premise underlying the social worker's investment in the study of his or her own practice or in combination with other practitioners is based on the "availability of information." The belief of the department's several administrators that social workers should examine their own practice is evidenced in their early support for one-page studies. The intent of these studies is to do "clinical data mining," drawing on what has been documented and reaching out to the provider for insights. The means to the study is the practitioner and it is he or she who will bring both interpretation to and recommendation from the findings. "Based on his/her clinical information cast in concepts derived from practice wisdom and done in partnership with a researcher, the findings simultaneously derive from and challenge the practitioner's interpretation—his/her reflection-in-action" (Rehr, 2001, p. xviii). The benefit to clinicians who engage in mining data is that they learn about their patient needs, about what has worked and what has not. Staff investment in studies bears out Ed Kilbourne's advice to physicians: "those caring for their patients shall themselves engage in studies, since not infrequently careful observations of patients yields lines of research which might be overlooked" (1988, p. 47).

For an administrator, practice-based studies are useful in many ways. They can inform about staff assignments and continuing education needs and report services to institutional administrators, regulators, the public, and support committees. When practice-based studies are done by social workers with other health care professionals, the results frequently are translated into multidisciplinary program changes.

A climate of practice-based study needs both administrative support as well as external resources. At this institution, the mining of data by clinicians and administration has been based upon a partnership in consultation and collaboration with practice-oriented researchers. The department has benefited from researchers who drew on practice-based research rather than on research-driven practice (Rehr, 2001). For this department, studies are practitioner- determined, following Jenkins' belief that "research findings must have utility for practice" (1990).

The staff and its administrators from its inception as a professional department have supported the need for analysis of social service practice and programs. It has modeled itself on the institutional belief that study enhances service (Williams, 1988). To date, over a period of fifty years, the clinical social workers, the social work division faculty, and its international scholars have studied and published over a thousand articles in peer reviewed journals (social work and other health care professions), in chapters, books, and in lay publications. It is these authors (and presenters at conferences) who attest to the enhancement of their practice and the programs that they serve and in social policy advocacy (Rehr et al., 1998).

AN ASPIRING RESEARCHER BEGINS AT MOUNT SINAI

Barbara Berkman, DSW
Helen Rehr/Ruth Fizdale Professor
Columbia University School of Social Work

It is difficult to believe that it has been over twenty years since I left my position as a researcher at Mount Sinai Medical Center. Had my husband not taken a position in Boston, I probably still would be at Mount Sinai today. This book, written by my former Sinai colleagues Helen Rehr (whose Chair, endowed in her name, I proudly hold at

Columbia University School of Social Work) and Gary Rosenberg, brings back my memories of the "heyday" at Mount Sinai, when interdisciplinary collaboration among the health professions was evident on every level—submitting grants, writing papers, and teamwork on the hospital floors. What an incredible and indelible experience this was for me. This book presents important memories for those of us who were there and great lessons for those who were not fortunate enough to "grow up" with Doris Siegel, Jeanette Regensburg, and Helen Rehr.

In 1962 when I joined the faculty of Mount Sinai School of Medicine as a young Columbia doctoral candidate, the Women's Auxiliary Board, the focus of this book's Chapter 4, provided "seed money" for this aspiring young researcher so that I could write my first of a series of grants which explored older patients and social work services. These intelligent avant-garde women believed that research was essential as the foundation for program development and that the information we would uncover could lead to enhanced services for patients. My early studies on screening and identification of older patients in need of social work services became the foundation of my research for over thirty years. I know that the board's early support for this pioneering work was not limited in impact to Mount Sinai. Eventually, the funding from this research were disseminated through publications and presentations throughout the country. This eventually led to improved services to patients in need of psychosocial help, as social work screening mechanisms became the norm for practice in most major hospitals. Today, as social work moves into community-based ambulatory care services, emphasizing primary care and ongoing health care management of chronic illnesses, we are bringing screening and case-finding into primary care. At the same time, we continue preadmission and admission screening for hospitalized patients' posthospital care needs so that discharge transitions can be facilitated more effectively. Thus the legacy of social work at Mount Sinai in this area continues.

Dramatic changes have occurred in patient care delivery, stimulated by advances in technology and new approaches to the financing of health care. Social workers in health care are still very visible, working as providers in new models of care. However, many of these new models operate as separate and fragmented entities, isolated from social support services. This raises our concern for the accessibility, efficiency, and comprehensiveness of health care service delivery. Thus, while we have had scientific breakthroughs, these advances do not necessarily carry equivalent provisions for the vulnerable and the economically disadvantaged. The pioneering outcomes of the Mount Sinai Social Work Department in developing programs for early identification of vulnerable patients in need of services, in the creation of patient service representative programs and employee assistance programs, in the commitment to health promotion and investment in interdisciplinary practices remain significant components of health care services. Continued efforts of professionals with vision such as Helen Rehr and Gary Rosenberg are needed today so that social work can be on the frontlines of health care practice, informing and addressing the needs of vulnerable clients who depend on our research, policy advocacy, program planning, and service delivery.

THIRTY-FIVE YEARS OF SOCIAL WORK AT ELMHURST HOSPITAL

Lawrence Cuzzi, DSW
Director, Social Work Department
Elmhurst Hospital

Any description of the Department of Social Work Services at Elmhurst Hospital begins with Helen Lokshin, who was the Director from 1964 to 1981. Her tenure predated the beginning of the original clinical affiliation agreement between the Mount Sinai School of Medicine and Elmhurst, which occurred in 1970.

This contractual affiliation was negotiated between New York City's Health and Hospitals Corporation and Mount Sinai to upgrade the quality of health care service delivered to patients. All physicians and senior clinical staff employed at Elmhurst were to be credentialed and employed by the School of Medicine, which would then be responsible for their professional performance and future training. Ms. Lokshin was included as part of that senior clinical staff as were six of the social work managers.

As the affiliation relationship matured Ms. Lokshin's interest in and experience with the elderly progressed to where she became an acknowledged advocate of providing specialized services to the geriatric population in general and more specifically at Elmhurst Hospital. This included social work intervention in their psychosocial life as well as medical care focused on their specific health needs. Her published articles attempted to highlight those services that would be needed by, at that time in the seventies, an underserved and little explored portion of our society.

This dedication was officially recognized in June 1982 when the Skilled Nursing Facility of Elmhurst Hospital was dedicated to her, honoring her advocacy and memorializing her commitment to the statement that "Our past is the link to our future." In 1982, Lawrence Cuzzi, DSW, assumed the position of director, which he continues to occupy to this day. The fact that there have been only two directors of the department in the thirty-five years of the affiliation underscores the common purpose of both Elmhurst and the School of Medicine. Such agreement allows the social work staff to concentrate on the mission statement to provide care to all citizens of the city, especially the new immigrants and the financially and medically poor of all ages, regardless of ability to pay.

Because of the inherent difficulty of providing such services to patients, especially with the usually low level of entitlements and resources, Dr. Cuzzi and his staff began to focus on two major issues in social work practice, namely, how to educate master of social work (MSW) students to work with this population and how veteran staff make decisions regarding priorities of social work services delivery.

With the vital support of the (then) Division of Social Work (Community Medicine) the department was able to explore the value of various methods of educating MSW students and also use the decision-making research to inform supervision of staff.

Nine articles were published in several refereed journals that enabled us to share this information with colleagues throughout the world. In addition, presentations were made at several national and two international conferences where the interaction with other social workers helped the department to deepen its understanding and use of the research results.

Current research is examining our involvement with childhood obesity and the innovative program established by our pediatric and child life staff to help both parents and children cope with this important preventive medicine issue.

At present, social work at Elmhurst continues to be an integral part of the health care service delivery. The number of staff has grown to over 150 MSWs, caseworkers, and other support staff and are found in every service within the hospital.

Social work leadership participates in the local chapter of the National Association of Social Workers (NASW) and the National Society for Social Work Leaders in Health Care.

One final example of the vitality of this department and its importance to both hospital and Health and Hospitals (HHC) administration is that of the eleven affiliations begun in the 1970s, Elmhurst is the only one where the senior social work managers are still employed by the affiliated medical school. This has allowed us throughout the years to attract and retain committed social work professionals who value the connection with The Mount Sinai Hospital and School of Medicine.

FROM EVALUATION METHODOLOGIST TO CLINICAL DATA-MINER: FINDING TREASURE THROUGH PRACTICE-BASED RESEARCH

Irwin Epstein, PhD
Helen Rehr Professor of Applied
Social Work Research (Health & Mental Health)

In 1968, having completed my MSW and putting final touches on my PhD in sociology, I left Columbia University for my first teaching position at the University of Michigan. Though the Midwest was no inducement, the social science-infused master's curriculum and prospects of future teaching in the doctoral program in social work and social science captured my academic imagination. From the start of my career, I was convinced that sociological theory and social research methods could contribute to social work understanding and decision making. There were few individuals and no other schools at the time that shared my perspective.

Though enjoying the intellectual stimulation that came from exchanging ideas with a "powerhouse" faculty, the painfully obvious lesion of my time in Michigan was that good social science was no guarantee of effective practice application. To illustrate: I arrived in

Ann Arbor during the Detroit riots. While Wayne State University School of Social Work faculty were providing services for displaced residents, some of my faculty colleagues in Ann Arbor were theorizing about whether it was the "lower-lower" or the "upper-lower" class Detroiters who were rioting and the grant possibilities inherent in this question.

Though ideologically uncomfortable, I prospered and quickly secured tenure and promotion. Nonetheless, I experienced a gnawing sense of frustration with what seemed like my own research irrelevance and the disdain for practitioners and social agencies that I witnessed among many of my Michigan academic colleagues. Practice wisdom was denigrated, and field placements were considered a pedagogical wasteland.

Taking a divergent path, with Tony Tripodi, I began writing for practitioners about evaluation methodology. We wrote some terrific articles and books together, well ahead of the evaluation movement, but the field was slow to respond, and, for all its college-town sophistication, Ann Arbor was not New York. I still wince remembering my discovery that the one "Chinese" restaurant in Ann Arbor offered "French, blue cheese, or Russian" with the complimentary iceberg salad. We won't even talk about the "Jewish-style" deli.

Today the restaurants have improved, but I am long-since gone. Alienated by the anti-agency culture of U of M, I returned to my source and took a job at Hunter College School of Social Work in New York in 1981. Hunter was known to be a practice-friendly and agency-oriented school and was just a short subway ride away from my beloved but sadly departed HooLok and the still-thriving Second Avenue Deli. But while the restaurants were cheap, housing costs were impossible on my Hunter salary, and my kids were in private schools.

Economic necessity and the desire to make more of a contribution to practice led me to evaluation consultation at various social work agencies when I was not teaching. My external evaluation efforts paid the mortgage, covered tuition, and brought me closer to practice, but what struck me most was that so few of my report recommendations were ever implemented.

Seeking a more direct integration of research and practice, I began a fruitful, twenty-year consulting relationship with Mount Sinai, the seeds of which were planted when I met Gary Rosenberg, then Director of Social Work Services at Mount Sinai. Our first meetings took place over doctoral dissertations when he was serving as an "outside committee member" for various Mount Sinai staff completing doctorates at Hunter. I loved the way his mind worked.

Both trained and applied sociologists, we shared practice-research perspectives in ways that were entirely unique in my prior career experience. Through Gary, I met Helen Rehr, that notorious deflator of academic pomposity, who became a cherished mentor, benefactor, colleague, and friend. Later, when Susan Blumenfield succeeded Gary as departmental director, she provided extensive support for my continuing work.

While the administrative support was unwavering, the nature of the work was changing. My early work involved helping individual and groups of Mount Sinai practitioners to do their own planning, monitoring, and evaluation research employing original qualitative and quantitative data that they collected with instruments they designed themselves. It was what I called "practice-based research," and this form of consultation became my form of practice.

Whether published or not, the studies that resulted addressed practice problems and informed programmatic decision making. However, they required considerable resources and start-up time, presenting problems of worker engagement and completion. Some studies faltered because of worker transfer or leaving the hospital altogether, one because the principle practitioner-researcher married the consultant. None enjoyed external funding.

Still, the projects were linked to practice questions posed by the practitioners themselves, and, when completed, they were much more likely to be utilized than externally conducted research. Even the ones that were not completed benefited from the conceptual work involved in specifying outcomes and conceptualizing interventions. However, they required departmental resources that were less and less available.

During that period, the National Institute of Mental Health (NIMH) started a program to support research center development in schools of social work. Thinking that Hunter and Mount Sinai might join together in securing one of these prestigious and sizable grants, I went to Gary Rosenberg, then Director of Social Work Services at Mount Sinai, and proposed that school and hospital explore this possibility. Such a center could provide much needed funding for conducting practice-based research studies at Mount Sinai and its affiliated hospitals and could employ Hunter faculty as research consultants to facilitate these projects. Gary thought it was a splendid idea and provided the initial funding.

In a spirit of total collaboration, I co-chaired that initiative with Ami Gantt, who was then the Associate Director of Psychiatry and Social Work at Mount Sinai. We began regular meetings with directors of social work from Mount Sinai and several of its affiliates—Bronx VA, Elmhurst Hospital, North General Hospital, etc. Health and research faculty from Hunter attended our monthly meetings, and we "hammered" out a proposal for a Hunter/Mount Sinai Practice-Based Research Center for Ami and me to take to Washington. It was not easy since some of my academic colleagues were quite vocal about their superior understanding of the needs of the field and their consequent conviction that they should set the agenda for the proposed center.

This was particularly ironic since the Mount Sinai department had a truly impressive research culture and a long tradition of publication. In fact, some of the Mount Sinai attendees at these planning meetings had more impressive publication records than some of my faculty colleagues. Ami and I decided that we would deal with them when we got the money and headed for Washington.

The response to our proposal was disheartening. NIMH program staff were not prepared for a jointly run center but had the greatest problem with the idea that practitioners would be conducting their own research projects. How could they be objective? Could their research be sophisticated enough to contribute to knowledge for the field? Could practitioners design and implement randomized, controlled experiments? What was the particular research theme of the proposed center? No, this was not what they had in mind.

Instead, they tossed us copies of successful applications submitted by the so-called research universities and sent us packing. Ami was in tears, and for me it was "same-old, same-old."

I remained undaunted however because I continued to see the knowledge-generating potential of working collaboratively with practitioners. Then, about ten years ago, I stumbled across a project possibility that transformed my work at Mount Sinai and opened a whole new door for my efforts at practice-research integration.

I had been asked by a team of Mount Sinai social workers and psychiatrists who screened candidates for liver transplant to help them design a prospective study to determine whether their judgments about who should receive a transplant were sound. Together, we explored different prospective design possibilities, quickly rejecting the notion of random assignment. At that point, I asked a question the answer to which was simple to them but was momentous for me—how many liver transplants have been done thus far in the department? The answer was close to 500. How many of these patients have you interviewed? Virtually all of them, was the reply. What intake information do you have about these people? All kinds of background information, psychosocial data, health data, etc. What outcome information do you have? Whether they survived the operation and how long post-transplant they survived. For how long post-transplant do you have this information? Up to three years.

Instead of designing a prospective study, I proposed a retrospective study conducted by the team, using the clinical information they already had. They accepted my suggestion, and we set about extracting information on every transplant conducted in the past five years. Social workers and psychiatrists began working as true colleagues, sharing theoretical insights, practice suggestions, and clinical recollections. In a relatively short time period, this became the largest, longest follow-up study of psychosocial risk factors and liver transplant outcomes ever done.

The project informed future practice and policy decisions and led to staff presentations and publications. The methodology employed was then proposed for a successful grant application to the National Kidney Foundation for a study of psychosocial factors and social work interventions with end-stage dialysis patients. This was followed by a grant from the Soros Foundation Project on Death in America for a study of a telephone support service for home carers of terminally ill patients.

I named this approach to practice-research integration "clinical data-mining" and gave a talk about it a few years ago in Australia at a conference honoring Helen Rehr. The subtitle of that paper was "mining for silver while dreaming of gold," and the implication was that I was well aware that these studies do not generate the kind of "gold standard" knowledge that evidence-based practice advocates continually extol. Nonetheless, they produce findings of real import to practitioners, contribute to knowledge for the field, and, most importantly, promote reflective, evidence-informed practice on the part of those who conduct them.

Since that conference, Susan Blumenfield and I have co-edited a collection of data-mining studies in health. Most of these were done at Mount Sinai. That was in 2001. More recently, Ken Peak, Daniel Medeiros, and I have co-edited a collection of clinical data-mining studies in adolescent mental health conducted by practitioners at Mount Sinai's Adolescent Health Center. That collection includes twelve peer-reviewed empirical studies on adolescent risk and counseling preferences by teams of social workers who had never before published anything or thought they could do research.

Correlatively, as a result of my continuing involvement in Mount Sinai's internationally focused Leadership Enhancement and Exchange Program, I've had the opportunity to collaborate with colleagues in Australia and Israel on practice-based research more generally and clinical data-mining in particular.

In fact, I write this about to embark on the trip to Israel where Gail Auslander from Hebrew University and I will be conducting data-mining workshops in hospitals in Jerusalem and Tel Aviv. In addition, my colleague Lynette Joubert from the University of Melbourne and I are currently co-editing a collection of multidisciplinary data-mining studies conducted by Australian allied health professionals.

Clearly my work at Mount Sinai has been central to whatever contribution to linking practice and research that I have made in my career. To my academic colleagues who are interested in effective research collaborations with practitioners, let me quickly restate my own practice guidelines that I set down for myself in 1993 but still work for me today:

- establish positive, trusting relationships based on mutual respect and appreciation;
- let practitioners set the research agenda;
- accommodate research concepts and techniques to practice norms and requisites;
- recognize practitioners' unique ability to contextualize, interpret, and apply research findings;
- employ active listening for concerns, theories, metaphors, and contradictions that surface;

- validate practitioners' desire to know and to reflect; and maintain a firm belief that practice-based, research-informed reflection will lead to more effective social work practice.

To my Mount Sinai mentors, supporters, and co-researchers, I can only offer deeply felt appreciation and a continuing eagerness to go down to the data mines again—together. There is more treasure to be found.

GOING ACROSS TOWN AND OUT INTO THE WORLD

Gary Holden, DSW

In the fall of 1990 I was finishing my dissertation at Columbia University. I was entirely focused on that process and not thinking very much about the next step in my career. Then, one day, Myrna Lewis, a fellow Columbia student and one of the best social workers I have ever known, said to me: "You should go see this guy I know at Mount Sinai." So I made the appointment, went out and bought a suit, and then went to my first appointment with Gary Rosenberg. It turned out to be the most important meeting of my life, leading to a life-changing fifteen-year collaboration.

After I became better acquainted with Mount Sinai and Gary with me, my role evolved into what I used to think of as a roving methodologist. As vice president of the Medical Center, Gary would match my skills with his and other health care professionals' interests, and then I would join their team to help to carry out a particular research project. Some of these projects were done in the Mount Sinai social work department and ranged from small practice-based studies (e.g., Mailick, Holden, and Walthers, 1994, on pediatric asthma) to larger scale department studies (e.g., Showers et al., 1995; Simon et al., 1995, on discharge planning). At the same time we initiated a series of practice-based studies at out affiliated social work department at Elmhurst Hospital. This research began with a study of the applied question of how workers prioritized admissions of high-risk cases when multiple high-risk cases were admitted concurrently (Holden et al., 1995).

Our group worked very well together, and so we moved on to a set of studies that asked if we can improve social work field education in hospital settings. Testing out Edith Abbott's idea of rotation, we presented the field with some suggestions for this core aspect of social work education (Cuzzi et al., 1996, 1997; Spitzer et al., 2001) and began a long-range program that continues today and is focused on developing social work educational outcome measures (Holden et al., 1996, 1997).

At Mount Sinai, outside of the Social Work Department we examined intervening with patients in the admissions office to lessen their anxiety (Holden, Speedling, and Rosenberg, 1992) as well as addressing issues on the larger profession (e.g., Holden, Rosenberg, and Showers, 1992; Rosenberg and Holden, 1997). We worked on large-scale health studies, including the Minorities, Risk Factors, and Stroke Study and the National Cooperative Inner-City Asthma Study (e.g., Holden et al., 1993; Wade et al., 1997).

The most dominant theme in this topical array has been technology. Shortly after I joined at Mount Sinai I began going there less. My ideal work day is sitting in my gym clothes at home in front of my computer, with my cats and my wife nearby, doing my work. Because Gary was more interested in product than presence, he agreed with me. I became a telecommuter and remained so until I left the medical school faculty in 1996. I would typically come into the hospital for half a day every two weeks or so for meetings and trips to the library. My position at Mount Sinai would have been near ideal for any new graduate—it was very active, very high-level health care and research, with extremely bright people and wonderful facilities. How often does a new social work researcher have the opportunity to learn from a social work pioneer like Helen Rehr as I have at Mount Sinai? Adding the ability to telecommute made it perfect for me, and I look back on that period of my life very fondly.

However, technology was also central to the themes of our work. For instance, we were invited in the mid 1990s to help Steven Spielberg's Starbright Foundation develop a technological intervention to help improve the lives of hospitalized children by connecting children in almost 100 hospitals throughout the United States. Although Gary and I were the only social workers on this project, it was our Mount Sinai team that developed and carried out a cutting edge series of randomized controlled clinical trials to test the effectiveness of this intervention for children (e.g., Holden et al., 1999, 2000, 2002, 2003). Although the intervention effects were small, we clearly demonstrated that this intervention reduced the amount of pain and anxiety experienced by the children who used it.

We began to think about the dissemination of research for practice long before the phrase *translational research* started popping up in government funding discussions. In 1993 we put together our first Gopher Resources for Social Workers package and then converted that to a Web-based resource as soon as the World Wide Web began to gain visibility (Holden, Rosenberg, and Weissman, 1995, 1996). This work morphed into the World Wide Web Resources for Social Workers (WWWRSW) site. This vortal was designed to assist social service workers throughout the world in obtaining the information they need from the Web. In its final version WWWRSW contained over 99,000 links and received 1,000 visits per day. We provided this service to social workers throughout the world for free for twelve years. Developments in the online world (e.g., Google Scholar, PsychExtra) made WWWRSW redundant, and we closed it down in January 2005. Beginning in 2002, we developed a professional news service—*Information for Practice* (IP). By the time it morphed into a news and new scholarship aggregation blog in January 2005, IP had attracted over 5,000 subscribers from sixty-four countries. The new IP service is located at http://www.nyu.edu/socialwork/ip/. Mount Sinai has a long tradition of service to the Harlem and East Harlem communities. WWWRSW and now IP continue in that tradition, but extend the focus to the entire world. Our most recent work in this line of research uses the tools of bibliometrics to examine the scholarship of social workers (Holden, Rosenberg, and Barker, 2005).

This rehashing of my past has been an indirect attempt to convey what an amazing opportunity I was given to develop myself and hopefully do a few things that have helped the field to move ahead. It is an opportunity for which I will always be grateful.

REFERENCES

Cuzzi, L. C., Holden, G., Chernack, P., Rutter, S., and Rosenberg, G. (1997). "Evaluating Social Work Field Instruction: Rotations versus Year-Long Placements." *Research on Social Work Practice*, 7, pp. 402-414.

Cuzzi, L. C., Holden, G., Rutter, S., Rosenberg, G., and Chernack, P. (1996). "A Pilot Study of Fieldwork Rotations vs. Year Long Placements for Social Work Students in a Public Hospital." *Social Work in Health Care,* 24, pp. 73-91.

Holden, G., Bearison, D., Rode, D., Rosenberg, G., and Fishman, M. (1999). "Evaluating the Effects of a Virtual Environment (STARBRIGHT World) with Hospitalized Children." *Research on Social Work Practice,* 9, pp. 365-382.

Holden, G., Bearison, D., Rode, D., Rosenberg, G., and Fishman, M. (2000). "The Effects of a Computer Network on Pediatric Pain and Anxiety." *Journal of Technology in Human Services,* 17, pp. 1-3, 27-48.

Holden, G., Bearison, D., Rode, D., Fishman-Kapiloff, M., Rosenberg, G., and Onghena, P. (2003). "Pediatric Pain and Anxiety: A Meta-Analysis of Outcomes for a Behavioral Telehealth Intervention." *Research on Social Work Practice,* 13, pp. 693-704.

Holden, G., Bearison, D., Rode, D., Fishman-Kapiloff, M., Rosenberg, G., and Rosenzweig, J. (2002). "The Impact of a Computer Network on Pediatric Pain and Anxiety: A Randomized Controlled Clinical Trial." *Social Work in Health Care,* 36, pp. 21-33.

Holden, G., Cuzzi, L. F., Grob, G. G., and Bazer, C. (1995). "Decisions Regarding the Order of Opening Multiple High-Risk Cases: A Pilot Study in an Urban Hospital." *Social Work in Health Care,* 22, pp. 37-55.

Holden, G., Cuzzi, L. C., Rutter, S., Chernack, P., Spitzer, W., and Rosenberg, G. (1997). "The Hospital Social Work Self-Efficacy Scale: A Partial Replication and Extension." *Health and Social Work,* 22, pp. 256-263.

Holden, G., Cuzzi, L. C., Rutter, S., Rosenberg, G., and Chernack, P. (1996). "The Hospital Social Work Self-Efficacy Scale: Initial Development." *Research on Social Work Practice,* 6, pp. 353-365.

Holden, G., Rosenberg, G., and Barker, K. (2005). "Bibliometrics in Social Work." Special Issue of *Social Work in Health Care.* Co-published as edited volume by The Haworth Press.

Holden, G., Rosenberg, G., Barker, K., Tuhrim, S., and Brenner, B. (1993). "The Recruitment of Research Participants. A Review." *Social Work in Health Care,* 19, pp. 1-44.

Holden, G., Rosenberg, G., and Showers, N. (1992). "Restricted Social Science at the National Science Foundation." *Social Work,* 37, p. 184.

Holden, G., Rosenberg, G., and Weissman, A. (1995). "Gopher Accessible Resources Related to Research on Social Work Practice." *Research on Social Work Practice,* 5, pp. 235-245.

Holden, G., Rosenberg, G., and Weissman, A. (1996). "World Wide Web Accessible Resources Related to Research on Social Work Practice." *Research on Social Work Practice,* 6, pp. 236-262.

Holden, G., Speedling, E., and Rosenberg, G. (1992). "Evaluation of an Intervention Designed to Improve Patients' Hospital Experience." *Psychological Reports,* 71, pp. 547-550.

Mailick, M., Holden, G., and Walthers, V. (1994). "Coping with Childhood Asthma: Caretakers' Views." *Health and Social Work*, 19, pp. 103-111.

Rosenberg, G., and Holden, G. (1992). "Social Work Effectiveness: A Response to Cheetham." *Research on Social Work Practice*, 2, pp. 288-296.

Rosenberg, G., and Holden, G. (1997). "The Role for Social Work in Improving Quality of Life in the Community." *Social Work in Health Care*, 25, pp. 9-22.

Showers N., Simon, E. P., Blumenfield, S., and Holden, G. (1995). "Predictors of Patient and Proxy Satisfaction with Discharge Plans." *Social Work in Health Care*, 22, pp. 19-35.

Simon, E. P., Showers, N., Blumenfield, S., Holden, G., and Wu, X. (1995). "Delivery of Home Care Services After Discharge: What Really Happens." *Health and Social Work*, 20, pp. 5-14.

Spitzer, W., Holden, G., Cuzzi, L. C., Rutter, S., Chernack, P., and Rosenberg, G. (2001). "Edith Abbott Was Right: Designing Fieldwork Experiences for Contemporary Health Care Practice." *Journal of Social Work Education*, 37, pp. 1-12.

Wade, S., Weil, C., Holden, G., Mitchell, H., Evans, R., Kruszon-Moran, D., Bauman, L., Crain, E., Eggleston, P., Leickly, F., Kattan, M., Kercsmar, G., Malveaux, F., and Wedner, J. H. (1997). "Psychosocial Characteristics of Inner-City Children with Asthma: A Description of the NCICAS Psychosocial Protocol." *Pediatric Pulmonology*, 24, pp. 263-276.

CONCLUSION

Recently the National Institutes of Health (NIH) and the National Academies of Science and of Practice recognized "the need for emphasis not just on medical intervention, but on the social, cultural, economic, family and community factors in prevention and treatment of health conditions" (O'Neill, 2001, p. 3). Recent work coming out of those supported by the NIH has recognized that cognitive counseling combined with medication is more successful in dealing with stress factors in individuals than medication alone. This recognition of the benefit of counseling speaks to a key place for social workers in diagnosis and treatment of individuals suffering stress. The difficult work ahead is to understand the counseling process. Donabedian (1973) noted counseling as the "process." However, it is known that problem and process are multifactoral and multisourced, while outcome is multidimensional. This suggests that governmental and health organizations see the need to move from their primary emphasis on laboratory and scientific research to integrate studies with those in the health care delivery systems. In order to capture the social-health and biopsychosocial factors that impact patients, families, and their communities, the research will need to focus on actual patients and their experiences with specific aspects of health care delivery, e.g., chronic illness, access, availability, health education and prevention, gender and cultural impact, and social ailments. In addition, who provides what to whom and of course the outcome and the costs and who pays must be on the study agenda.

While social science and behavioral research may be the "gold" standard, it is more than probable that data mining will prove valuable. The documentation of clinical social workers' interventions along with the chart entries on behalf of those in need and receiving services have demonstrated the value of social workers in enhancing practice and institutional programs. The major challenge facing both medical entities and social work research enterprises is to rapidly translate findings into improved patient care. When all is said and done, studies that affect social work practice and policy will require a practitioner-researcher partnership.

Chapter 8

Community Medicine and the Social Work Connection

> Social work at Mount Sinai represents not only a vital and essential component of the present Community Medicine effort, but in spirit and in fact, it represents the first tangible expression of our institutional commitment to understand and respond to community health needs. (Dana, 1983, p. 11)

In 1968, when the Mount Sinai School of Medicine of the City University of New York was created, it committed itself to a social and community focus as well as to the clinical and biological missions of modern medicine. The philosophy was one readily committed to by Dr. George James (a former New York City Commissioner of Health and one concerned with the health of communities) as the school's first president and dean. Dr. Hans Popper, Mount Sinai's leading pathologist, conceptualized the community as the third factor in medicine alongside biology and clinical practice (Niss and Kase, 1989).

The Department of Community Medicine chaired initially by Dr. George James, the appointed president and dean, was followed by Dr. Kurt W. Deuschle as chairman of the new department. Dr. Deuschle had headed the first such department in a medical school at the University of Kentucky. Dr. Deuschle described his work: "the task of Community Medicine, as evidenced at Mount Sinai, is first to identify health problems in the community by epidemiological techniques, and then to link resources in the Medical Center and other health institutions in East Harlem and bring them to bear on the community's most urgent problems" (Bosch and Deuschle, 1989). The Department Of Community and Preventive Medicine (as it is currently named) forms an important bridge between the specialized services and the people outside who need these services.

Community medicine's role is a new one in medicine. We are interested in more than medical care; our concerns are the total health problems of communities. Some of us are doctors with traditional backgrounds in clinical medicine and the public health disciplines, but we are also nurses, social workers, nutritionists, medical economists, medical sociologists, and statisticians. (Deuschle, 1970, p. 97)

Deuschle projected a concept of community medicine as a multifaceted professional and scientific approach to identifying health needs in the community and developing and testing new programs to meet those needs. Knowing the community and translating Mount Sinai to the community were the first tasks of the new department. Social work, from its inception, had been active in the community and was prepared to participate in the team effort to affect the mission of community medicine.

Social work was given a key position in the Department of Community Medicine along with the more traditional resources of epidemiology, biostatistics, health economics, population-based health sciences, health care delivery planning, the behavioral sciences, and environmental and occupational medicine.

BACKGROUND

The Jews' Hospital, initially a social service hostel, changed to The Mount Sinai Hospital in 1868. Over time, the hospital moved from its charitable base of servicing the "needy sick" to that of a medical institution guided by a medical and lay leadership. From the hospital's beginning, the wives of the supporting Jewish philanthropists sought for a humane and social perspective for the institution (see Chapter 4). An auxiliary board was formally created in 1916, and it has continued its social commitment to the hospital.

Massive immigration and the progressive movement set the stage for social work to develop and provided some outstanding and creative individuals with an opportunity to make distinctive contributions to social work's growth (Austin, 2000). The voluntary not-for-profit sector was developed by religious and business leaders, and the growth of social sciences and the interest in applying social sciences to social problems along with the establishment of women's colleges helped found the field of social work. Social work in health care benefited from collaboration at the earliest stages of its development when Dr. Richard C. Cabot organized with Ida Cannon the social work department of the Massachusetts General Hospital in 1905. However, differences occurred between social scientists and social workers in both education and professional development, and a separation resulted. In 1916, Harvard ceased offering social work courses and replaced them in 1921 with a department of social ethics headed by the same Dr. Richard Cabot who had helped to formalize the place of social work in health care practice. This division forced a separation between the study of social problems and the application of solutions. It is a distinct advantage that recently at Mount Sinai the divisions of social work and of behavioral science were combined into a single division: Division of Social and Behavioral Sciences and Social Work. The Edith J. Baerwald Professor of Community Medicine (Social Work) continues as chairperson of the division.

Over the many decades, the social work department's professional leaders worked in close alliance with the auxiliary board, both of which brought a humanitarian focus to services given within the institution. Each brought something special to the other. Social workers helped to bring an in-depth perspective to medical care and to the auxilians. The auxilians supported socially oriented programs. Social work focused on how both illness and the care offered will influence "the patient's and family's course for good or bad" (Bosch and Deuschle, 1989). As the professional and lay groups worked together dealing with issues of health care delivery and the need to affect change and lobbying for quality care for all, they influenced the trustees, administration and physicians to value a social-health model of care versus the traditional medical model. The early social mission of the Jews' Hospital was broadly interpreted into a comprehensive social-health center of care offered by a multiprofessional health care staff to the residents of its local community and to those who sought its services. The contributions of social-health services to the institution's diverse users were in support of the hospital's Judeo-Christian social mission. The alliance of the social work leaders and the auxiliary board members had gained a key place in the institution.

Thus, as a medical school was in plan, in the late 1950s and early 1960s, it was evident that social work would be included in its design. In the 1960s society was undergoing major changes—a consumer movement, women's rights, patients' rights—that were recognized as affecting the delivery of medical care and influencing the need to rethink medical education. The 1950s and 1960s seemed to call for a new kind of doctor. The traditional emphasis on biomedical knowledge and technology was not enough. The recognition that medical care was affected by health needs, patients' rights, doctor-patient interrelationships, and a host of other social-environmental factors led medical schools to look to a "community medicine"—a "community health"—a "social medicine" approach. Thus, a third faculty was created "as a component of modern medical education, together with the basic science and clinical faculties" (Dana, 1983). Social work with its clinical skills, its focus on community organization and development, its ability to reach out to the local residents, block associations, church organizations, other health, and social service providers and its interprofessional collaboration with medicine earned social work a place in the new academic center.

Initially social work sought its own department as a discipline within the academic medical center, to stand alongside other departments. An alternative view was to situate social work in a department that supported multiple disciplines and professions with an overall service, educational, and community focus. The argument was made for the latter, and social work became a partner with other disciplines in a department of community medicine. In addition, social work was seen as critical in joining with other professions in addressing population issues in communities. Thus, social work with its clinical and community-networking skills and its demonstrated ability to enhance institutional services was included as a major partner in medical education, and a division of social work in the department of community medicine was created.

The board of trustees and the auxiliary board had supported this initiative, which was further helped when the Aron family (long-time supporters of Mount Sinai) established the Edith J. Baerwald Professorship in Community Medicine (Social Work), the first Endowed Chair of Social Work in a medical school in the United States. The three consecutive holders of the chair have served initially and concurrently as directors of the department of social work services (Appendix II). Today, the Baerwald Professor and chairperson of the division, a social worker, was a former director of the department. The position of the director of the department is separate from that of the academic division chairperson (by circumstances and not by design). The current director of social work services holds an associate professorship in the medical school, along with the joint position of associate director of the hospital.

THE DIVISION OF SOCIAL WORK

A division of social work was founded in the department of community medicine and joined with other divisions: behavioral sciences, environmental medicine and occupational health, epidemiology, health economics, and international programs. Social workers in becoming faculty members of community medicine complemented the traditional educational components of basic sciences and clinical services. Social work's roles in research and in education—in medicine, social work, and the other health care professions and groups—were allocated to the division. In its history the majority of its educational and study enterprises was and are still undertaken by the clinical staff in the department of social work services. A number of these practitioners hold faculty positions in the division in addition to their clinical and administrative positions at the Mount Sinai Hospital. The Mount Sinai School of Medicine has a number of affiliate institutions whose programs are utilized in medical education and in multiprofessional studies. A number of these affiliated social workers have also been inducted into the division faculty. As faculty members, social workers serve on a range of committees, including admissions, appointments and promotions, and curriculum. Social workers are also active in the policy determinants of the school.

The focus of community medicine is to give "both form and substance to the social mission of modern medicine" (Bosch and Deuschle, 1989, p. 461). One of its focuses is on the community—its social-health problems, its needs, the resources available, program enhancement, coordinating services, the financing of health care, and the assurance of the availability and affordability of services for the people in need. There was a good fit between social work's emphasis on the community, its belief in advocacy for social change in policies and laws, and its activities in creating a network of social and health agencies to provide services to families and their members and to persons in need or at risk for health and social problems. What social work lacked, community medicine provided. It reunited the more objective and descriptive social sciences with social work, provided the economic theory and analysis lacking in social work education, and provided a grounding in epidemiology and population-focused practice.

SOCIAL WORK ROLE IN MEDICAL EDUCATION

The doctor-patient partnership was a key educational component of the division's curriculum. Social work has an important role in medical education within the medical school. Throughout the history of the medical school the social work faculty has been part of curriculum planning efforts to enhance the humane and caring aspects of medical practice, to teach a multidisciplinary practice, to teach effective interviewing, to help students and faculty understand the multiple cultures and beliefs represented by the population of persons served by the medical profession, to understand how social risk affects medical risk, and how to deliver community-based services directed toward populations at high risk. It has planned and participated in required epidemiology and biostatistics courses, in introduction to medicine, and in interdepartmental teaching in preclinical and clinical courses, and it provides faculty to the newly created two-year course for first- and second-year students titled "The Art and Science of Medicine." In this course, social work and behavioral science faculty serve as instructors teamed with medical faculty colleagues to provide a rich experience in applying medical and social-environmental understanding of diverse people and their health and illness and to learn the assets and problems of how services are delivered.

During the third year of the curriculum, in the Community Medicine clerkship, a social worker codirects with a physician on student projects dealing with health care delivery, the organization, financing and evaluation of services, the epidemiology of given health problems, the social and economic costs of illness, and the biopsychosocial and cultural factors that influence health and illness behaviors. The clerkship teaching roles fall largely to social workers in the department of social work services. The Medical Center and its school provide a curriculum emphasizing collaborative skills and health promotion and education within the complex intricacies of a health care system and its funding. A disease-specific focus is interwoven with a supervised hands-on experience in the many services of the hospital.

In its educational roles in community medicine, social work brought a social-health perspective into all of the professional health care students' classrooms. In collaboration with their colleagues, the emphasis was to

- understand the community's social-health status;
- identify health and social needs, the gaps in service, and the programs essential to meet them;
- optimize availability and accessibility of services;
- draw on social-epidemiological methods to screen for vulnerable populations and provide primary prevention;
- contribute to social-health planning efforts;
- further the community's understanding of public policy as it affects funding and service delivery;
- create a network of social-health service to allow for comprehensive care, including the use of information. (Rehr et al., 1998, pp. 129-157)

To these educational objectives, the social work clinician-faculty introduce their students—medical, social work, others—to the community and to the families of patients in their homes. They enlist the community as their partners in education (Peake et al., 1998).

Social work assists in educating medical students in the significance of the contributions of other disciplines associated with the delivery of social-health care and in medicine's collaboration with identifying population needs, understanding the impact of the psychosocial factors of an individual and family lifestyle on medical compliance, coping with the economic and social costs of illness, identifying the vulnerable, and financing health care delivery. Social workers in their teaching role with students help them to identify a social-health problem, study it, do a literature review, analyze the data, and offer recommendations. With the Community Medicine Fellows and residents in preventive medicine and occupational health, social workers participate in curriculum development and in interdivisional seminars that deal with the biological, psychological, and social-environmental factors that affect individuals who are ill and their families (Rehr and Rosenberg, 2000).

This department in its clinical work with its clients recognizes that academic social work does not fully prepare its students for work in today's health care settings. Thus an in-the-field experience is integrated to develop the clinical base. To be efficient in a health care setting, social workers need to have a specialization that is both health and mental health directed. This requires a knowledge of the multiprofessional nature of health care and the collaboration with other health professionals in order to serve clients.

> To function effectively in health care practice settings, social workers must have current knowledge of the health care delivery system and must understand dynamic changes in the system and how to deal with them. To practice effectively—they must understand the intricacies of organization structure, health care financing and its correlation with service delivery, and the financing of hospital settings. [They need] knowledge of disease, disorders and disability—and their impact on individuals, families, society and themselves. (Rehr and Rosenberg, 1984, p. 106)

The department and the division fulfill this objective.

Recently the department of community and preventive medicine introduced a family practice course codirected by a social work faculty member and member of the department of social work. It also created a PH program for medical students, house staff, fellows, faculty of the school, and for those in the community interested in public health. Social work faculty serve as course directors and offer elective courses and thesis advisement. Through their faculty appointments in community and preventive medicine, well-qualified community social workers provide education, supervision, and mentoring to medical students, house staff, and fellows in such departments as pediatrics, psychiatry, and anesthesia.

SCHOOLS OF SOCIAL WORK

The division has formalized key relationships with several New York–based schools of social work to offer master's degree students, and others, a field practice experience within the five Mount Sinai affiliated institutions. Under the leadership of the department and the division, social work has forged a major relationship with a School of

Social Work in developing a social work academic-practice partnership model for the education of social work students (Caroff and Rehr, 1985). The model has gained cross-country interest. At the same time, a number of Mount Sinai social workers have been active in an adjunct faculty relationship with the interested schools. This social work model also offers postgraduate educational opportunities within the medical school's Brookdale Continuing Education Institute for members of all professions, as well as advanced social workers, so as to introduce new knowledge, enhance skills, and teach how to assume accountability responsibility.

Faculty in schools of social work who are active in teaching health and mental health practice and policy are encouraged to apply for appointment in the division to provide some teaching and research collaboration with the medical school faculty. Currently members of the faculty of five schools of social work hold an affiliate appointment in the Mount Sinai School of Medicine. The relationship is a mutually rewarding one where the richness of both medicine and social work affects the teaching and learning of both professions.

COMMUNITY PRACTICE

The department of social work services had played an active role in relating to its East Harlem community since before the beginning of the Model Cities Act. Social workers had related to consumers of health care by engaging in a wide array of community agencies. With lay participants' goal of enhancing consumerism in contributing to the assessment and advocacy of quality health services, they joined with others. Drawing on a range of opportunities to reach consumers, they joined in active membership in community agencies and began writing for journals, books, popular magazines, and newsletters. The intent was to raise awareness in and to empower the consumers of health care. Recognizing that a medical center and its professionals, programs, and services must be responsive to those who live in the region, the department undertook a key position in assuming a partnership with its local residents (Peake et al., 1998). It adopted the principles enunciated by McDermott (1969) and supported by the Medical Center's boards of trustees and administration:

A university medical center must permanently concern itself with two groups of people, not just one. It must concern itself with its traditional constituency, the individuals who see its help—and it must concern itself with its community, which may or may not be immediately adjacent to it, and which contains at any one time—far more people who are well than are not.

Doris Siegel, when she was invested as the first Edith J. Baerwald Professor Community Medicine (Social Work), put the commitment succinctly, "We must reach out more aggressively not only to those whom we serve, but to those whom we should serve" (Siegel, 1969, p. 2). With regard to the commitment to those who crossed the threshold for services, the department initiated a Patient Representative Program to deal with obstacles including fragmented services and barriers to care and to uncover gaps regarding needed programs. In pioneering this "ombudsman" program for the hospital's clientele, the social work staff advocated on their behalf. At the same time, the department developed social health advocates, a trained group of aides who brought an essential culture awareness to dealing with local residents. Both programs continue, with an expansion to include the hospital's neighbors and others who are in need of learning of and securing entitlements due them. Today REAP (Resource, Entitlement and Advocacy Program) is an active storefront service for those who need help and referral, and it advocates for improved community social and health services.

Social work is active in community planning and holds community organizational memberships on behalf of the institution. In that process, a director of community relations serves the institution along with the department of community medicine in relation to its local communities. The director of community relations, the current director of social work services, and a past founder and department director serve on the medical center's community board. These hospital social work leaders bring a special understanding to the board in regard to community social-health needs. They support the community leaders, support their social-health planning efforts, assist them in grant writing and in seeking funding, and serve in linking programs to enhance services to community residents. The social worker, director of community relations, serves as a bridge between the operational and academic enterprises of the medical center and community groups. Good community relations and partnerships that involve the community as equal partners are crucial for conducting research, particularly for those at risk in the community for poor health and disease. Medical researchers at Mount Sinai rely on division faculty to provide for their entry into the community and to help them forge effective partnerships with relevant community organizations. Social work faculty serve as members of the East Harlem Health Planning Committee and have provided leadership on projects such as building housing for the elderly of East Harlem and in programs for the prevention of heart disease through increasing exercise, smoking cessation, and changing eating habits that lead to poor heart health.

RESEARCH

The research efforts of social work tie it closely to community medicine. Social workers in the beginning decades of the twentieth century were employing epidemiological methods to learn of the impact of social, environmental, and occupational conditions on local community residents. Surveys and epidemiological studies are intrinsic in community medicine research. Social workers were quick to undertake such studies. In the latter half of the twentieth century, the division with the work of the department's clinical staff have studied and written about how to enhance several key areas:

1. the department's service to those in need;
2. a cost-effective service base;
3. the social-health care efforts of the institution;
4. multiprofessional collaboration and partnerships for the improvement of service;
5. social work's role in medical education;
6. social work in its own professional educational roles; and
7. a lay-consumer and professional partnership for enhanced services (see Chapter 8).

As the university medical center developed, it recognized that it had two major constituencies to deal with. It had that group of persons who crossed the threshold for help and it had its community at large, local or distant, including those groups who may or may not use the institution. With both constituencies, social work made major contributions—via its clinical skills, its home- and school-based programs—it offered direct services and studied the delivery of care so as to enhance it in the community; and it developed partnerships with organizations and groups so as to undo barriers for needed services.

The division faculty developed expertise in investigating the psychosocial consequences of drug use, protective and resiliency factors in minority youth, and at-risk behaviors through a family interaction perspective and in understanding violent and abusive behaviors in family members; all these projects were supported by the National Institute of Drug Abuse. The division faculty also provided research building capacities, with Fogarty support to other places, in Argentina, India, and South Africa. The department faculty also provided leadership in AIDS research and in researching services for the mentally ill. These efforts were also supported by various governmental agencies.

CONCLUSION

In being members of a faculty within a faculty in community medicine in a medical school, social workers have benefited from that association, as well as contributed to a multiprofessional collaboration in medical and social work education, services, and studies. It has moved the medical model of care to a transition of care in a social-health delivery model. Social workers have been influenced by the community's health status in population needs terms. They have learned how health care is fiscally supported; how social work in medical settings is financed; how to incorporate cost-benefit services and accountability; and how to assess social services in relation to clients served. As social workers in a community medicine faculty, they have learned from their interactions with their health care colleagues from epidemiology and biostatistics to assess populations at risk, to enhance the study of process and outcomes, to understand the significance of prevention and health promotion, to engage in a community-based collaboration in the planning and delivery of service to the residents, and to join with others in the promotion and support of sound social-health policy. For social workers in health care, their active roles in community medicine have helped them to recapture the clinical relationship with society and with specific populations and their social-health needs in addition to direct service to patients and their families.

Niss and Aufses, in their book on the history of the Mount Sinai School of Medicine, describe the contributions of the division as follows:

> The faculty members of the Division have conducted clinical social work and behavioral science practice and research in the Medical Center and its affiliates on a wide range of subjects. The concept of population at risk has involved social work and behavioral science faculty in such diverse studies as research on the needs of the elderly in East Harlem, factors predictive of child abuse, the relationship of social support to ethnicity and culture, the longitudinal examination of drug abuse, smoking and violence, and numerous other projects geared to primary and secondary prevention. Through research, the Division contributes to new knowledge of the social and psychological costs of illness and the impact of illness on the social functioning of individuals and families. (Niss and Aufses, 2005, p. 204)

Chapter 9

The Globalization of Social Work Services in Social-Health Care

AN INTERNATIONAL EXCHANGE AMONG SOCIAL WORK LEADERS

During the last quarter of the twentieth century, the world moved toward more togetherness and accessibility. Industries, particularly the large American ones, became global, and a number of nations became more cooperative with one another and also more competitive. The rise of an international perspective had both positive and negative outcomes. In some instances, internationalism collided with nationalism—threatening global stability, unrest, and even war. In other instances, it brought a Western perspective to the developing countries, which absorbed change very slowly and with discord. However, in making the peoples of the different countries more accessible to each other, it also made them more aware of each others' social-health problems and needs.

As one views the social-health problems in Westernized countries, it is apparent that the problems are similar, albeit their severity, priorities, and services may differ. Hunger, poverty, homelessness, malnutrition, and dislocation do exist in the West. These problems also exist in developing countries with an inexorable impact on the health status of and on the lack of medical care for their people. The media is rife with articles describing the woeful plight of large numbers of persons in these countries. Sickness is ubiquitous, and illness is neither age nor gender based; they are prevalent in relation to environmental conditions, poverty, turmoil, starvation, and individual behavior. The lack of available resources is common knowledge, despite the yeoman effort of the nongovernmental agencies' (NGOs') attempt to stem the hemorrhaging situations. The government support for services to meet the social-health needs of the people is scarce.

The United States is not without a major measure of social-health problems among its people. A shift from government support of social programs for the needy to that of charity and faith-based organizations has affected the availability of resources. At the beginning of the twenty-first century, the United States had over 44 million of its population either uninsured or underinsured for health care in any one year. Currently, more than 82 million people do not have health insurance coverage during any two-year period of time. Children make up a large part of this number. Vast numbers of the elderly unable to pay the skyrocketing costs of needed medications go without, and they are reported to do without essential nutrition as well. One of the wealthiest nations in the world is not meeting the needs of the vulnerable. In the less developed countries, the problems are more dire. While the NGOs are attempting to meet known needs, their resources are limited, and frequently the provision of their services is controlled by the local government and selectively administered. Where there are some resources available, persons who are needful are unprepared and uninformed in how to seek relief.

It is essential to address these needs by those in the helping fields. In the opinion of the authors, what is a "must" is a level of leadership that is not only knowledgeable about the community's needs but is committed and skillful enough to gain the support of the needed constituencies who will advocate for resources. To exercise social work leadership in a medical institution requires a mission and ability to see beyond prescribed areas of responsibility so as to sense opportunities for enhanced service programs. Such a leadership must adapt services and the understanding of (the agency's) purpose to changing needs and resources. Skilled social work leaders are able to focus on both physical and human resources, finding innovative ways to confront changing needs within the institution and within the community served by the institution.

The program of an international exchange of social workers was developed on the premise of the principle of enhanced leadership. It is critical that leadership in an organization should have the attributes essential to secure direct services for its clientele. Also it requires the skills to facilitate enhancements of programs in relation to the recognized needs of the population served. In general, the usual progression to leadership in an agency is for clinically experienced staff to move to supervision and to administration often with little or no management training. There are situations where directorial appointments are made from outside the organization. However, in the social work field 90 percent of those who reach administration do so from within (Berger, 1993, p. 8). While some may have an inherent capacity to lead, most administrators in social agencies need to learn and develop managerial skills.

The hospital setting is one of the most complex, with its multidisciplinary environment and with the cultural diversity of the population it serves. Effective leadership requires an in-depth understanding of the institution—in a system sense—and knowing its employees and the support sources. It also requires a recognition of the clientele served and to be served. An ability to relate to the multiple networks within and outside the organization is fundamental. Knowing one's own operation is a must and requires measurements to demonstrate its efficiency and effectiveness to its various constituencies. In a multidimensional setting such as the hospital, one needs to make one's service visible and be able to market both institutional and social services. Also it is essential to create a climate of challenge and motivation among the staff and to have adaptability and flexibility to deal with changes and constantly improving regulations and innovations. This requires leadership skills.

Can there be gains from an exchange among those who manage social work programs on the international scene? The question was posed by two regional sources of social work in health settings—in Israel and Australia. Social managers on exchange visits to America and American visitors to both countries highlighted the social-health problems common to all three countries. We hypothesized that the ability to adapt changing environments and client needs is one of a myriad of leadership skills that can be enhanced by comprehensive leadership programs with the institution and by drawing on the experience, diversity of ideas, and innovation of colleagues and peers at home and abroad. Cross-cultural exchange among social workers can help expand their views of local, regional, and national health needs and issues, thereby broadening and enhancing leadership opportunities and skills. Such an exchange can provide leaders opportunities for comparison, analyzing differences and problems, exchanging ideas, and observing programs that serve comparable needs.

THE ENHANCED LEADERSHIP PROGRAM

With recognition that urban problems have multiplied and that some social programs continue and some contract, social workers in a few Westernized countries sought to exchange ideas and methods with the intent to enhance services for those vulnerable groups in their own areas. A program of shared experiences and educational opportunities for social work leaders was established by the department and division of social work in New York (at The Mount Sinai Medical Center), with the key social workers being in Israel's cities of Tel Aviv, Jerusalem, and Haifa and in Australia's cities of Melbourne, Sydney, Adelaide, Tasmania and Canberra. The program followed visits to both Israel and Australia by Mount Sinai staff. Those visits to social work service programs revealed that they were also facing economic crisis and experiencing similar concerns. Albeit expressed in local terms, issues of access, quality, evaluating service, developing services, and management were voiced along with a wish to be exposed to other social work programs grappling with similar issues. The development of an international social work education exchange between Mount Sinai Medical Center and key social workers in health care organizations in Israel and Australia supported the notion that Western social workers from different parts of the world, facing comparable social-health problems, can learn from each other, but only if ideas and "methodologies are selectively adapted" (Midgley, 1990, p. 297) so as to allow for regional and cultural differences. In sharing content and experiences where objectives are comparable, knowledge and practices can be adapted to meet social-health needs of given populations within the context of respective government policies and expectations.

The program created in 1988 with the Israeli participants and in 1990 with the Australians continues to date. Israel, Australia, and the United States were suffering from an explosion in costs of medical care, with their economies, while markedly different, stretched to their limits. Cost controls had already been imposed in each country, and more controls were sought to curb expansion and to reduce expenditures. Given the fiscal crisis each was undergoing, there was with it a view to cut what were seen as "nonessential" or even "luxury" programs.

As we have become aware, across the oceans, of the growing social-health needs of more people and of the gaps in services, a public demand for more comprehensive, integrated, and individualized care in a social-health context has grown with the need to demonstrate that social work can provide such care in quality and cost-effective ways. What was evident was the need for information to offset the poor or unclear public perception of social work and the lack of know-how to demonstrate its effectiveness. Each country registered its domestic concerns about access barriers to services, more so in the United States than in Israel or Australia (but, in the latter two, in particular for Arabs, Bedouins, and Aborigines), plus limited community support services (again more so in the United States), and the need for outreach. On the professional side, fighting off turf invasion, enhancing collaboration, making social work visible, and recurring social work mobility and status in the health care field were repeated concerns in all three societies.

The objectives of the project that were agreed upon by all principals at Mount Sinai and abroad were "to enhance leadership capabilities, to enrich each other in the knowledge and skills needed for the implementation of quality programs in the service of people, to be able to assess current programs, to contribute to their improvement, and to draw on and conduct applied studies to generate relevant information so as to be able to offer recommendations for social-health policy with the ability to translate to cost-effective service programs" (Rehr, Rosenberg, and Blumenfield, 1993, p. 20).

The means outlined were to review programs, initiate and engage in an exchange of what works and what does not for individuals and their families with given social-health problems, and determine how to achieve beneficial and cost-effective services.

It was assumed that leadership skills could enhance the services offered to an institution's clientele. The premise was that "a social work leader must adapt services and the understanding of [the agency's] purpose to changing needs and resources" (Rehr, Rosenberg, and Blumenfield, 1993, p. 13). The responsibility of social work leadership was to focus on resources and ways to deal with changing needs and availability of care within the institution and the community served.

During the 1980s, economic difficulties were prevalent enough to recognize the jeopardy to programs serving the needy, as well as the possible survival of the profession of social work. The fiscal crises crossed countries, and it was apparent that social workers were asking a number of questions that touched on the continued viability of their services.

- What is needed; are all in need being reached?
- Are social work services beneficial to those served?
- Is the social work system in health care efficient? How can it be managed effectively?
- Are services cost-effective? How can cost-effectiveness be demonstrated?
- How can the value of service be communicated to clients, to key others: administrators, regulators, etc.?
- How can quality and accountability be assessed and demonstrated?

An Enhancement of Leadership Program (ELP) was discussed in 1986 following visits to Israel's health care programs and then to select cities in Australia by members of the Mount Sinai Social Work Department. Social work services in hospitals were at a low ebb at that time of financial stress. All over, questions were being raised about the continued availability of services for those at social-health risk. The critical concerns dealt with the viability of social services and with the conditions and resources social work leaders considered essential for their continuance and support. The issues were discussed across geographical areas—in Israel, in Australia, and here, at home. It was apparent there were more similarities than differences in the problems each faced. "Access to social-health services, safeguarding quality of care, reaching those in need on a timely basis, developing required services, and ensuring the availability of essential resources and their cost-effectiveness, efficiency and quality management" were the common concerns (Rehr, Rosenberg, and Blumenfield, 1993, p. 24). Cultural, political, organizational, and fiscal factors were the differences among these exchange partners.

In recognizing the similarities of their problems, they identified the areas they wished to consider:

1. "professional accountability and quality service delivery;
2. a knowledgeable way to gather and use information and data;
3. the need for skills in program assessment, followed by program planning; and

4. the ability to offer and demonstrate beneficial and cost-effective services" (Rehr, Rosenberg, Blumerfield, 1993, p. 16)
5. the ability to affect public policy and enhance administrative program planning.

These were skills required to serve individuals, the system, and social-health care providers. The exchange program attempted to solicit the specific areas of each group as each perceived the vulnerabilities of services. Surveys and exchange among the participants uncovered the need for skills in "management, developing and marketing social-health programs, enhancing staff performance, and developing professional accountability" (Rehr, Rosenberg, and Blumenfield, 1993, p. 18). In addition, all participants sought program evaluation skills—what and how to gather information and how to use data; the ability to do needed applied social-health studies and consumer and staff satisfaction studies; to enhance collaboration among responsible partners; and to identify priority needs.

The three-month exchange, twice a year, for four exchange scholars (two Israeli and two Australians) offered opportunities to senior social workers to view problems and programs in New York City, to observe their effectiveness, and to discuss applicability to the home needs. The visitors described their own programs—the positives and the negatives—with the local social workers. While the exchange was essentially on a "Western" perception of services and practice, the focus was on leadership needs and problem solving and also on the clients and clients' needs, along with their own roles in their institutions and agencies. The means was a curriculum relevant to their requests, which dealt with a literature content, observation, hands-on experience in areas requested, a study approach to an area of concern, and open discussion on issues identified.

The key concerns raised as a result of needs assessment given to prospective applicants to ELP were (in no particular order of priority):

1. Managerial skill, including assessment of existing programs and planning for new services.
2. Evaluation of staff performance: measurement tools, assignment and coverage determinants, motivating long-term staff, and adequate orientation of staff.

3. Undertaking quality assurance in service delivery, and professional accountability.
4. Staff recruitment and staff development skills (continuing education), including individual and group supervision.
5. Conducting needs assessment, and use of information gathered.
6. Enhancing collaborative skills for required interactions.
7. Undertaking applied social work studies for program' enhancement, and for interpretation with relevant others; fundraising projects.
8. Developing leadership abilities for hospital and medical care interaction.
9. Consumer-oriented programs, self-help and networking with consumer organization movements.
10. Planning for patients' rights, patient representative programs, and ethics committees.
11. Developing a partnership between the field and academia.
12. Enhancing group service skills.
13. Developing a contractual problem-to-outcome approach.
14. Chart documentation.
15. Teaching medical and social work students.
16. The enhancement of social work services in a range of specialized practice arenas, e.g., Oncology Services, Adult/Pediatrics, Rape Services, Abortion Services, Employee Assistance, Adolescent/Teenage Services, End-Stage Renal/Transplant Services (Rehr and Epstein, 1993, pp. 79-93).

The curriculum was based on the expressed interests of the visiting scholars. The Mount Sinai Task Force developed a curriculum that included bibliographies, procedural manuals, scheduled assignments, group discussions, and a "hands-on" experience individualized to the participants' expressed interest. Each scholar worked with a range of staff members and with an individual mentor. The curriculum was focused on enhancing leadership abilities. The emphases were on

- administrative and managerial skills in fiscal management, accountability for services, program development for social work and social-health care, allocation of resources, quality of care

and cost-effectiveness assessment, and participating in intramural social-health policy and decision making.
- Marketing social work services by making them visible and understandable, demonstrating their benefit, and communicating benefits to appropriate others.
- Program evaluation by gathering and utilizing information in partnership with relevant participants, making recommendations, implementing essential change and reevaluating feedback (with staff).
- Developing collaborative and cooperative skills at different levels of objectives.
- Developing professional accountability measures to include standards and indicators of service delivery; a uniform management information system, documentation of services rendered and problem-outcome or other acceptable measurement tools to permit cost-benefit review.
- Developing applied social-health studies relevant to services to targeted population (e.g., frail elderly), and utilization and consumer and provider satisfaction studies.
- An in-depth examination of related service programs, e.g., alternate level of care, geriatric social services, psycho-educational treatment model, health education and patient representative programs (Rehr, Rosenberg, and Blumenfield, 1993, p. 22).

The objectives of the project were

> to enhance leadership capabilities, to enrich each other in the knowledge and skills needed to implement quality programs to serve people, to be able to assess current programs, to contribute to their improvement, and to draw on and conduct applied studies to generate relevant information in order to offer recommendations for social-health policy with the ability to translate to cost-effective programs.

Were these objectives achieved? It is risky to claim outcomes from a three-month exchange of senior professional social workers. Evaluations on their exit from the program indicated learned content and general satisfaction. It was after their return to their home bases and over a period of time that reports came back in letters, in publications, and in presentations in forums about the impact of the experience. They cited what they referred to as "bringing it back" in journal articles in which they assessed the experience:

- The enhanced position of the field of practice in relation to academic social work;
- The establishment of a strengthened health sequence in the schools of social work;
- A strengthened position for social work leadership in their institutions and among health care providers;
- Social work leaders were participating and contributing to social-health policy deliberation both within the institution and on a regional basis;
- Enhanced intraprofessional and interprofessional collaboration;
- The development of an information system; the use of in-house data and studies to promulgate for program enhancement; the introduction of accountability-measures, patient satisfaction surveys;
- Departmental studies to enhance services and cross-agency networking;
- Their involvement in new program development, projects, primarily inter-professionally designed;
- Their own professional self-development including presentations at forums, and in first-time publishing of programs e.g., disaster preparedness, rape crisis programs, respite care, emergency trauma services, enhanced interviewing skills (Soskolne, 1993; Irrizarry, 1993; Haywood, 1993).

As to the Mount Sinai social work staff involved with the visitors, they reported that the ELP "helped them to learn about their own as well as the visitors' practice and programs—to reevaluate [their] own clinical work as well as programs (Rehr and Epstein, 1992, p. 91) and to negotiate for needed change.

All exchange social workers involved in the project (to date) come "with high levels of motivation, skill and relationship to peers—ongoing evaluation reflects an increased level of awareness of institutional and departmental leadership skills, and skills which translate into meaningful projects and programs" here and at home (Rehr and Epstein, 1992, p. 92).

The international ELP has led to several other gains:

- for all involved, a recommitment to professional identity and social work values;
- for a number, advanced studies for professional enhancement and career development;
- an exposure to "survival strategies" for clients and for the profession;
- an enhanced practice-academic partnership;
- activated roles in professional organizations;
- an international colleague-hood;
- the introduction of comparable educational programs by Australian graduate social work scholars to other country social workers (e.g., Hong Kong, Thailand, Singapore);
- the creation of the International Conference on Social Work in Health and Mental Health—triennial conferences held to date in Jerusalem, Melbourne, Tampere, and Quebec. All have attracted social work practitioners and academics from around the world.

The international exchange among social workers is a modest example of cooperation and sharing of experiences and learning. In dealing with the similarities and the difference in the needs of the respective populations served by their social-health agencies, social workers learned from one another. Opportunities to examine programs and to think resources and results have allowed these "exchange scholars" to stand away from the immediacy of the pressures of their own programs and to rethink goals and creative problem solving. Becoming engaged and informed in an exchange among social work leaders, researchers, and practitioners resulted in new lessons and ideas. All involved challenged themselves as to whether they could evaluate and reshape their programs. They argued about the impact of fiscal constraints and the ongoing demand on their workers and their services. They cited the impact of the serious social ailments of AIDS, substance abuse, person abuse, violence and accidents, malnutrition, accidents, and unintended pregnancies. Compounding these ailments was the recent impact of terrorism on unprepared localities. As they deliberated, they drew from each other different experiences and ideas, and in that cross-cultural exchange the social workers viewed local, regional, and even national social-health needs and issues. The exchange offered opportunities to compare situations, to analyze differences, to exchange ideas, and to observe programs within institutions and in different communities. They also identified areas in which they thought the ELP could be enhanced. All returned home still having to face limited resources and to deal with safeguarding services. Yet, all wished for a continuing exposure to what other social workers in other countries were facing and doing.

The local in-house staff participants reported their experience as one of the best continuing education opportunities and as a mirror of their performance, allowing them to refine their thinking in regard to their own practice, collaboration, and participation of studies. They also commented on the exposure to other cultures, systems of health care, and the comparability of professional social work in Western countries.

One limitation of the program is that the opportunities for exchange are available to only a limited few. It was apparent to all the principals in Israel, Australia, and in New York City that means would need to be developed to broaden the base of the exchange experience—in essence to strengthen the at-home investment. Three major areas have been in discussion: one deals with the role "graduates" can undertake with peers in Israel and in regions of Australia to advance leadership potential; the second deals with what the future direction of the project should be to accelerate leadership enhancement opportunities; and the third is what should the field's present role be with the schools of social work in order to secure advanced education in leadership development.

THE NEEDS OF DEVELOPING COUNTRIES

All participants noted that irrespective of country of origin, resource and health problems are critical policy and program issues. Social workers in Westernized countries are concerned about these problems in developing countries. Also in many places, local workers have tackled these issues regionally and in some instances at the national policy level. However, they have limited experience and resources in dealing with the extent and impact of poverty and hunger and the consequences. Over the past ten years, social workers have met in international exchanges where shared experiences have connected them to understanding and dealing with comparable problems. The third world countries face unique economic situations that have impeded the development of available social-health services. Basically, it's a problem of accessing health care. The resources and the number of trained practitioners are limited. Health care services appear to be outside the purview and understanding of the "medical" systems prevalent in many of the developing countries. Indigenous (traditional) medicine is culturally based and tends to be more affordable and accessible than conventional (Western) medicine. However, both are considered as essential in caring for those in need. It has been acknowledged by those who have encountered the "indigenous" practices that there is a need to invest in developing professionals who can be leaders in contributing to social-health policies, develop accessible programs, and train other practitioners. Dealing with the prevailing beliefs and cultural attitudes requires an indigenous group of practitioners (Parks, 2002).

Working at the local level, international social workers and NGO staff have introduced indigenous practices in an attempt to allow the people to reach needed medical services and even food stations. There are a few westernized social workers who have adapted their community organization and development knowledge to the local situations in developing countries. They have drawn on local citizens to advocate in their own interests. Their methods are directed at community residents, involving them in the local issues of illness and care, hunger and food programs, and health maintenance. Midgeley (1990) notes that "Third World countries can learn from the West, if methodologies are selectively adapted to local conditions" (p. 297). She also believes that the experiences in third world countries can contribute to Western social work programs. Indyk (pending publication) in describing her experiences in Argentina and India maintains that a "bottom-up" approach to dealing with social-health needs can create programs to serve those in need while also training health care professionals to be invested in relevant social problem solving. She highlights that the indigenous worker is the key player in problem-solving activities. Similarly McKay et al. (2004) have demonstrated the effectiveness of a community development approach with local residents in small communities in South Africa and with residents in the South Bronx, New York.

The experiences of ELP scholars have led them to propose a program that could be helpful to workers in the developing countries.

They are responding to the calls for help in what would be a cultural, regional approach to local residents to secure needed services. They have projected an International Institute for the Enhancement of Social-Health Services to be created by the partners of ELP to offer personnel training, service development, and simple assessment opportunities. Candidates would be social workers, NGO employees, and other social-health care providers (anywhere) who seek a time-structured experience in programs that deal with marginalized and/or needful persons to improve their access to social-health care. Over time, as personnel is developed via the exposure to selected programs, they foresee a coalition of social workers and others who will have "graduated" from the Institute and who will make available their resources to other international social workers and NGO workers who express needs.

THE NEEDS OF WESTERN SOCIAL WORKERS

Another project in the planning stage that also arose out of the ELP experience is the International Educational Institute in Social-Health, which is a joint research venture among the social work sectors of universities in selected foreign countries and in the United States. This project will establish an international partnership among the schools of social work and selected major centers of health care, teaching, and research. The purpose is to remedy the lack of application of study findings to both social-health policy and programs. Students and staff from one educational setting will be educated in interdisciplinary programs, undertaking studies and being exposed to studies in social-health issues, and will learn how to apply the outcome to the identification of key regional and cross-national social-health problems of individuals, groups, and specific populations. Once past the initial period, we foresee that other university schools of social work and academic medical centers will replicate the program.

The model for creating partnerships between higher education institutions and major health care delivery centers and teaching and research centers will integrate practice and research via education. It will offer

- a model for the future of the development of leadership in health care with an international thrust toward social-health policy and programs;
- a model to train graduate students and current practitioners in the assessment of programs and policies for the enhancement of patient/family services—in an interdisciplinary setting;
- a model to create a strong connection between academia and service to bridge the gap between them; and
- a model that is cost-efficient in that it trains both students and practitioners concurrently, with students fulfilling needed credits and practitioners achieving enhanced skills.

OTHER ENHANCEMENT OF LEADERSHIP PROGRAMS

It is difficult to evaluate the effectiveness of the enhancement of leadership programs; however, subjective assessments by participants affirm the value of the exchange. The model for enhanced leadership confirmed the benefits of gaining direct experience, including exposure to strong leadership at academic and service/research levels, in a major multidisciplinary service setting. The program includes hands-on learning by doing and exposure to theory both in the classroom and through the dynamic exchanges of American, Israeli, and Australian ideas and experiences. Opportunities to create other cross-national exchanges help social work leaders broaden their views of their local, regional, and national health needs. As leaders join together to examine social-health problems and policies, ideas and programs are cross-generated among them and modified to the local cultural needs. Such an exchange provides leaders and those involved in the program

- an insight in their appraisal of comparable problems in their own locale;
- opportunities to compare programs and discover gaps in services;
- increased awareness of parochialism, status issues, and turf battles, placing them in proper perspective;

- opportunities for an international perspective, an understanding of social and health problems, and their impact on people in different regions and of the resultant global tensions;
- opportunities to understand the more meaningful cultural factors that influence communication, negotiations, and, ultimately, decision making;
- opportunities to see the similarities and differences and to explore each other's experiences and perceptions of needs and resources to deal with them.

Leadership is not a genetic characteristic. It is learned, developed, and enhanced. This program has demonstrated that a curriculum based on the expressed needs of a group of experienced practitioners facing comparable service delivery and fiscal support concerns, and implemented by a senior staff of clinicians and administrators in an institution strongly supportive of teaching and research within its service programs, can enhance leadership capacities in all participants.

The gains from the ELP and the International Conference, both of which continue, and from the proposed International Institute (for developing country social service personnel) and the International Educational Institute would be a coalition of international social workers and other health care providers in a multiprofessional exchange of knowledge and programs. A cadre of localized but internationally based social-health leaders in cross-national opportunities would be available to review community social-health problems and the means to create tomorrow's leaders who would provide and plan services, regionally based.

Chapter 10

Medicine and Social Work: The Social-Health Challenge

The health care field is changing. Its delivery patterns are in flux. While doctors try to retain the values of the doctor-patient relationship, social workers in health care seek to find safeguards for the social-health needs of increasing groups of ailing and vulnerable people. As the delivery services shift, the funding of care changes, the population increases, and the technology of medicine is enhanced, social work in health care is challenged to move from its traditional in-hospital services to patients and families in order to be responsive to their needs amid the many changes in social-health care. The twenty-first century has been visited with a multitude of advances in medicine, yet the advancements are not without problems. Economic, societal, and political events have impacted health care, leaving Americans without an equitable social-health policy. The "right to health" for all, a principle held in the mid-twentieth century, was passed over for the principle of "the right to health care" for Americans. Neither is currently available.

In the nineteenth and early twentieth centuries, society dealt with the effects of the Industrial Revolution and the diseases resulting from crowded slum conditions, poor work situations, lack of sanitation, pollution, and exacerbations of urban living. Public health measures, antibiotics, regulated safety standards, drug and food quality standards, campaigns against lifestyle abuses, and the explosion of information were a few of the advances of the last century to foster the health of the populace. In addition, the federal government (with regional support programs) introduced a host of legislative directives to support the sickness, disability, and health needs of a range of different population groups while contributing to expanding the hospital bed capacity across the country and supporting the education of health care professionals. Industries were supportive of their employees' health status as both employers and employees negotiated coverage for medical care and for wages lost during absence from work due to illness.

The twentieth century reflected remarkable gains in scientific innovations and in social-health supports. The most effective as far as the general population is concerned were the public health contributions affecting water, air, and environment with their resultant disease eradication or reduction (Thomas, 1977). These measures, along with rehabilitation programs affecting injured soldiers introduced during the wars, projected the significance of the biopsychosocial effects of disabilities on individuals and the need to assist with them. The incredible achievement of all these contributions was that life expectancy advanced about thirty years from forty years of age in the first part of the century to seventy-eight years at its end. This is a remarkable gain, but not without consequences.

THE ECONOMICS OF HEALTH CARE DELIVERY

The benefits of those prior years are fast being eroded. The fiscal crises and a resulting public conservatism at the end of the last century have flowed into this century affecting health services and leaving the public without an adequate social-health policy. The major changes in health care delivery have occurred over the last twenty years. There has been a shift from a voluntary health care system with its public and private social-health support to a commercialization and corporatization of services. Rising hospital costs and the fragmented health care financing system have put vulnerable patients at risk for access and care. Hospitals are in financial difficulties and need to be made viable once again (Davis, 2004).

The individual has become more directly responsible for the cost of health care. Increased premiums, larger deductibles, and reduced government and employer support of services have shifted a rising level of medical costs onto the individual for his or her own and for family coverage. The growing numbers of unemployed have lost health care coverage, requiring self-coverage of premiums or no health coverage at all. Employers are increasing cost sharing or dropping health care coverage for their employees. Medicare patients have begun to encounter physicians who are closing their practice to them due to marked cuts in reimbursement and delays in payment for services by the government agency. Today there are over 44 million persons uncovered for health care, almost two-thirds are employed but are considerd "the working poor," and over 10 million are children. At some time during any two-year period more than 84 million people are not covered by health insurance.

The predominant values that influence today's health care delivery system are based on market decision making and the concept of shared responsibility. In earlier and perhaps more liberal times, shared responsibility existed among government and the voluntary (charitable) sector to provide employer-employee benefits and insurance in some combination for underwriting costs of care for individuals and their family members. In those times, care for the ill was responsive to both personal and community needs by federal provision (The Model Cities Act of 1968).

Current commercial decision making has impacted the principle of community support for both voluntary and government sponsored health care. As voluntary hospitals are taken over by commercial health organizations and they adopt a dollar-driven bottom line, there is a separation of institutions from the communities they were originally planned to serve. In addition, industry, by claiming fiscal crisis, has moved to cut employee benefits for health care, imposing a larger responsibility on the worker for coverage.

The support service has lost some of its meaning, and the notion of "community" has given way to a "corporate" survival mode for most voluntary hospitals. In many cases charitable not-for-profit organizations that formerly shared in assisting those in need have found themselves with diminished resources and in fiscal difficulty in continuing to support their past pattern of services, and many have reduced services to those with limited or no health care coverage.

When the federal government shifted payment for hospital stays for Medicare patients, it triggered the development of prescribed lengths of stay based on diagnosis, affecting the entire hospital/health care industry. The advent of diagnosis-related group (DRG) payment for a patient's hospital stay was intended to control inpatient stays, eliminating unnecessary stays and thus to control their cost. In eliminating the traditional per diem reimbursement, which paid for a hospitalization period without jeopardy to institutional reimbursement, it closed the door on longer stays without medical necessity as prescribed by the DRG. The implementation of DRGs fostered shorter hospitalizations, shifting to ambulatory care for many patients. One result was that it led to hospitals caring for a greater volume of sicker, seriously ill patients instead of the former pattern of a case mix. The impact of a primarily severely ill hospitalized group of patients placed a greater demand on hospital personnel than when hospitals had cared for a patient mix and their needs. Currently, many persons who leave the hospital need further at-home supports. Those services tend to be in short supply except for those who can afford them. Families are absorbing the increasing burden of care of their sick members, adversely affecting work productivity and economic growth. While shortened hospital stays may reduce the cost of hospitalization, the introduction of new technology and the growing demand for service have not reduced the overall cost of illness. The direct and indirect costs to individuals and families who support the "at-home" needs of discharged "sicker" patients are affected by major social costs to them (Ancona-Berk and Chalmers, 1996). One perceived benefit of an early DRG-related discharge is that patients are most responsive to healing in familiar surroundings, which tend to be more supportive than those of the hospital (Simon et al., 1995).

The government also developed the Resource-Based Relative Value Scales (RBRVS). Its implementation is intended to control the costs of physicians' services. As implemented, it has created winners and losers among the different specialist groups, resulting in increased conflict among physicians and confusion in the paying population. There has been an increased demand for talented business management skills for both hospitals and doctors to deal with the changing reimbursement patterns for health care services. This new type of administration deals with negotiating, contracting, and management, drawing on marketplace strategies. The current business climate in health care services has resulted in a national scrutiny of costs and lengths of stay for similar diagnoses given in the different regions of the country. It has led to protocols of standards and care affecting their payments. In a number of regions it has resulted in a form of "rationing" of services for different groups.

THE NEW MILLENNIUM

In the new millennium one can expect scientific advances that will affect medical care for individuals and will affect their lifestyle. The field of genomics will be responsible for a new focus on gene-related disorders. Knowledge about genes and their functions will contribute to the knowledge of disease and how the body and health are influenced by them. New drugs reach the marketplace almost daily that affect physical and mental pain and that modify disease-related conditions. Technological advances have already touched the surgical suites, resulting in the use of minimally invasive ambulatory surgery rather than surgery that requires inpatient stays. The benefits can be remarkable, but some can be problematic. Innovative rehabilitation procedures have given new ambulation potential to many, but, for the most severely disabled, there is the need for supportive care. Some predict that an antiaging drug will be developed in the near future—allowing the elderly population to extend life perhaps another twenty years (Bloom, 2001), while others predict a longer life but with chronic illnesses. Information technology will markedly change individual care delivery. It has already affected the way in which baby boomers inform themselves about their health and illness (Mellor et al., 2004), generally without professional consultation.

With all the projections of scientific gains and innovations in medicine, the social-health problems of the 1950s remain prevalent today. The uninsured sick, the homeless, immigrant populations, and those suffering poverty and hunger are daunting concerns. Chronic illnesses are not expected to go away; in particular, arthritis, hypertension, heart disease, and diabetes will continue to pose health and financial problems. Severity of illness impacts the individual and his or her family in functional and attitudinal ways. Present-day professionals have limited training to deal with the social costs of chronic and progressive illnesses to families. Mental health problems will continue as evidenced in present-day living patterns. It is estimated that one in five adults suffers from depression, anxieties, stress, and fears that affect the quality of life. Societies, in both the less developed countries and in the Eastern world, are not without epidemics of flu, malaria, dysentery, even tuberculosis. The latest onslaught on innocent people is the increasing number of terrorist attacks, and more are projected.

None of the gains comes without challenges and costs to individuals, families, and the population. The means by which people seek medical care and how they receive it have changed. Medicaid and Medicare are the federal and state means to support the medical care of low income sick elderly and disabled individuals. In the new millenium as the fiscal crisis remains unresolved, the states have begun to cut their Medicaid assistance to given groups, joining the federal government in its reduction of payments to hospitals for their care of Medicare patients. The states differ in their support of drug benefits to the needy elderly and disabled. Insurance companies have followed government patterns and also have tended to reduce reimbursement rates for hospital services (Rehr and Rosenberg, 1986, pp. 84-85). The recent legislative act to deal with the skyrocketing costs of prescription drugs for Medicare beneficiaries appears to have serious limitations. While supporting medication costs for the eligible poor, medication costs will still remain under pharmaceutical determination and will include a prohibition to purchase drugs out-of-country where they are cheaper. The new legislation does not assist the elderly and/or disabled to meet their medication needs at reasonable levels. The fiscal crisis has affected the health care system in its ability to provide available, accessible, and comprehensive care. The burgeoning numbers of HIV/AIDS patients and the large numbers affected by social ailments, e.g., violence, substance abuse, have made severe demands on a failing system.

Already on the horizon is the growing population of the elderly, with the ailments of chronic diseases requiring acute and long-term care. Baby boomers will soon double the number of aging persons, many of whom will require social-health care for chronic illnesses. While the baby boomers tend to hold the belief they will not suffer the illnesses that their parents have had, the medical experts continue to predict that the chronic illnesses of the cancers, cardiac disorders, and diabetes will be in their future as well (Mellor and Rehr, 2005). Irrespective of the beliefs of baby boomers about their projected aging health and economic status, the social-health care providers do foresee the need to address key issues that they anticipate in both the short and long terms. They acknowledge America's health care is changing. It is in a state of flux.

Population demographics such as the vast number of current elderly and the number of baby boomers will impact a health care system that is unprepared to cope with the anticipated demand. The latter has begun to ask what their health will be like; what services will be needed; what will be available and accessible; will quality be safeguarded; who will provide what is needed; will they be knowledgeable, and how will care be paid? Given the current climate of economic uncertainty of a deregulated and commercial health care market, of curtailment in employer-employee benefits, and in government and insurance cost containment practices, it has become more and more difficult to be assured of the quality and accessibility of today's services, let alone project for tomorrow. Among the most critical concerns are

- the growing inequities in health services, in particular, access to care not only for the millions of uninsured and underinsured, but also for those covered by commercial insurance, as well as those who encounter governmentally capped services;
- the epidemic of social disorders, including the range of abuses (substance and person) as well as violence, accidents, and suicides;
- the growing number of social ailments such as cirrhosis, emphysema, AIDS, and obesity from lifestyles and from behavioral, environmental, and work conditions;
- the ailments resulting from homelessness, poverty, and hunger, which undermine health and people's timely use of health and social service facilities and other support services;
- chronic illnesses and disabilities, which require complex social-health measures;
- the impact of a fragmented health care delivery and a fragmented payment system;
- those functionally limited (physically, developmentally, socially) who are at home or placed and require multiple social-health support services;
- the present-day limited and noncoverage of preventive and health maintenance services;
- the limited and inadequate availability of community social-health resources;
- the social costs resulting from at-home and family-supported services, placing greater demands on patient and family resources;

- the continuing impact of stressful, anxiety-based living and work conditions on growing numbers seeking help with mental health concerns;
- the growing use of information technology to deal with medical and social-health conditions, while eschewing professional consultation; and
- righting the balance of resource allocation between public health and the medical care system.

These key issues will affect the vulnerable, who will need preventive, medical, and social-health assistance. Today, they continue to be in need. Tomorrow, the increasing numbers, as the population grows, will further impact the medical and social-health resources. While medicine has tended to be the approach of many to deal with the problems noted above, the trend is changing. More people turn to information services such as the Internet for consultation and suggestions regarding their social-health problems, leading to self-doctoring. In addition, there has been a proliferation of self-care and self-help groups, frequently without professional guidance. Also there has been a rise in nonprofessional personnel entering the counseling, support, case management, and fringe health services, providing additional therapies—some of which may be beneficial but most are untested, nonsupervised, nonregulated enterprises based on prescribed dieting, exercises, and behavioral modification, costing billions of dollars to a worried, stressed, and anxiety-ridden public. The impact of specializations in medicine has contributed to the fragmentation of services and lack of coordination of patient care. The rising cost of health care has impacted vast numbers of Americans, and the fragmented financing system has affected the viability of hospitals.

SOCIAL WORK AND SOCIAL POLICY

For all the progress social work has made in health care over the last few decades in its ascendancy to leadership to top administrative levels of a number of medical institutions (Rosenberg and Clarke, 1987), and in facilitating the shift from a biomedical model to a social-health and people-oriented focus to medical care (Rehr et al., 2000), the gains are receding as the health care crisis continues. However, in its recent past, it is important to recognize that social workers in hospitals promoted the enhancement of institutional services by helping to make them user friendly, e.g., ombudsman and patient service representatives, by broadening the patient base via outreach programs (Rehr and Rosenberg, 1986), by fostering motivational and coping capacity to deal with the impact of illness, by assisting patients and families to secure support services in their homes following hospital discharge (Simon et al., 1995), and by increasing satisfaction with the services (Showers et al., 1995). Physicians and nurses joined in a multiprofessional approach to secure a social-health model of care as they witnessed the safeguarding of treatment goals for patients and the enhanced capacity of social workers in diagnosing and bringing comprehensive patient-family assessments to care.

As one examines the achievements over the past fifty years, social work in health services has placed its concentration on improving the service delivery to hospitalized patients and their families. Medical social services were lodged primarily within the medical institution, supported by the government policy of incorporating payment for social work services for inpatients in need. The focus of social work services was largely on individual and family biopsychosocial dynamics and on environmental factors affecting the illness and the patient's coping with its impact after hospitalization. The traditional system facilitated social workers to find those with social-health needs via their coverage of assigned areas and/or by referral from health care professionals, primarily doctors and nurses, by other service providers in the community, or by patients and families. By the end of the sixties social work developed its own case-finding system and was no longer dependent on others (Berkman et al., 1980).

While social work achieved a collaborative partnership with other health care professionals in the hospital, the fiscal crisis furthered a conservatism regarding the "right to health care." The introduction of deregulation of care and its privatization and the increasing corporate milieu in governing health care delivery added to the confusion and chaos in the health care industry. It produced uncertainty and even conflict among the different disciplines as payment for services became more restrictive. There was clear evidence that existing piecemeal social-health policies and attempts to "add on" by Congress would not resolve the impediments. The prevailing emphasis in the American health care system was on "who will pay for what." It was essentially provider and payer oriented—hospital and doctor focused—with the payment formula being service based. The patient is on the receiving end of a care based on episodes of treatment!

Social work services are prescribed in Medicare as a service component to inpatients; but funded allocation for the service is hospital administrative based. Thus, it can range from one worker to a number irrespective of bed capacity and can predetermine ambulatory programs irrespective of patient needs. Medicaid is state determined, and social services are provided based on the fiscal status of the state, i.e., more or less, again not determined by need. Some insurance companies have included social work visits in their clients' coverage. Also, change in hospitals due to financial pressures have resulted in shifts from a centralized department/division structure to a program and patient unit administration, resulting in decentralization affecting the staffing of social work services (Berger et al., 2003).

There is no public social-health policy for maintaining health and supporting well-being. Social work has played a limited, if any, role in promoting public social-health policies—unlike its earlier position in social reform movements in the beginning of the twentieth century. In an earlier publication the authors raised a series of questions that they believed needed to be addressed:

> Have rising costs of health care played havoc with our ability to plan and reach sound public policy? Have we bypassed an essential care policy for Americans by over concentrating on institutions and providers? How has commercialization and deregulation of health services affected access and quality for individual care? Should health care be cost controlled? Should American policy support a "right to health care"? Are hospitals social utilities for the common good, or private enterprises? (Rehr and Rosenberg, 1991, p. 112)

The health care debate has spilled over from the last decade of the twentieth century into the new millenium. The issues of today are similar to those of yesterday. They remain lodged in cost, quality, fragmentation, availability, and accessibility. The health care scene has worsened. Hospitals (their programs), physicians' services, and those of other health care providers encounter dramatic changes as a result of the attempts to control costs and the expansion of the commercialization of care. Much is related to the government's ongoing reduction in reimbursement rates allocated to special programs and in the programs of managed care and health insurance companies. The hospital scene has begun to resemble corporate enterprises responsible to their shareholders for profit making as against their past status as a public social utility. Regional hospitals are merging or affiliating to achieve cost efficiencies. They are downsizing staffs; have reduced and/or eliminated nonprofitable services; shifted from a case mix of inpatient care (except for the most severely ill) to ambulatory care; and now provide episodic rather than comprehensive care. There is a projection of a mix of professional, paraprofessional, and self-help services, confusing to public users, as providers tend to engage in multiple functions, previously maintained by others with minimal (if any) educational supports. Compounding the chaos is the introduction of an Internet porviding health care diagnostic and therapeutic services, which are used by individuals who self-medicalize or are just curious. Much of this information is given by promoters of care without licenses or certification and thus accountable to no one.

Twenty years after the development of an accepted social-health model of care was considered valid for the American public, this model of care is being curtailed. Yet the current issues in health care that require a social-health direction and public understanding and involvement remain:

- the impact of chronic and progressive illness and the need for a continuum of social-health care;
- those diseases relevant to the aging process, their prevention and health maintenance;
- the recognition of the interrelationship of diseases to social and environmental conditions and advocacy for environmental changes;
- the impact of the increasing emphasis of market forces and their effect on available and comprehensive care and/or medical services, as well as their cost;
- the recognition of the costs of social-health care as a component in reimbursement;
- the need for ongoing evaluation of the outcome of health care interventions in the context of both physical and social functioning;
- the perception of the role of families (in both an informal and formal context) in the support of those who are ill and patients

seeking more responsibility for decision making in the health care;
- education for quality end-of-life decision making and the sound use of palliative care so as to achieve a good life and a good death;
- the more than 45 million Americans without medical insurance, who are mostly minorities, as well as low-income employees without or with limited benefits (the Commonwealth Fund, cmwf.org/newsroom);
- educating the public in prevention and health maintenance and how to be informed users of health care services;
- assisting individuals who utilize nonmedical sources (Internet) to deal with their ailments by becoming adequately informed;
- advocating for available and comprehensive care for the mentally and cognitively impaired;
- educating health care providers and the public on the value of a model of social-health care;
- developing a public-provider partnership for accountability and needed enhancement of services;
- recognizing the locus of health care in ambulatory and emergency services and in the community in selected settings.

These are the critical social-health issues with which health care professionals and the public must deal. A study undertaken by the New York Academy of Medicine, with the support of the Hartford Foundation, identified a number of these health care trends that warrant major shifts in the social work curriculum so as to affect social work services (Volland, 2001).

As has been noted, American health policy has been focused on the medical factors as offered by the providers, the institutions, and their medically related payment means. The future requires a social-health policy that is based on people-related needs and an informed public as to the quality and effectiveness of what is available to them (Rehr and Rosenberg, 1991, p. 112). There is something awry in a health care system that leaves over 44 million American uninsured and almost that number underinsured. The burden of caring for these people when illness and disability strikes falls on the covered population and on institutions and providers with limited resources to provide adequate care.

TOMORROW'S SOCIAL WORK

What has been suggested is that the current health crisis leaves social work in health care with an uncertain future (Pecukonis, 2003). As both practitioners and administrators of social work services in medical institutions, we agree that health care delivery systems are in change. We believe, however, that social work has made contributions in conceptualizing and assisting in the implementation of a social-health model of services and that it can redefine its roles and contributions to public social-health policy and to social services to those in need. The public and the providers have experienced the benefits of a comprehensive social-health care model, and, if advocated for by the public, they will continue to promote it.

Social work has begun to shift from its traditional role with hospitalized patients and their families in discharge planning. While it will continue to be available for such services, its work with inpatients will be in supporting diagnostic assessment and in counseling to optimize treatment and aftercare. The financing of medical care has shifted to outpatient arenas. Therefore, social work in health care will need to take place in the community while continuing to serve the hospitalized patient. However, social work services will need to be covered payment entities. Social work will be both individual and family needs focused and also active in assessing the needs of given populations. Social work's past experience promotes a concept of a "continuum of care" for those with chronic illnesses and long-term needs. As it contributes to the knowledge of individual and population needs, it assumes defined roles and functions within a multiprofessional service team. Drawing on one model of care (Kotelchuk, 1992), social work's functions are lodged in the projected paradigm in Figure 10.1.

Currently many medical institutions, and the academic medical centers in particular have assumed a commitment for the seriously ill. This includes a concentration on tertiary care patients, which draws

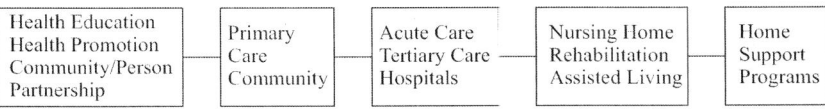

FIGURE 10.1. Social Work's Functions

on specialists for diagnosis and treatment. Except for serious exacerbation in the illness, the majority of care is currently lodged in ambulatory services. Ambulatory surgery has been an early shift from hospitalized surgery. The trend has fostered the development of an innovative class of physician-hospitalists. This hospital-employed group assumes the responsibility for the hospitalized patient for both diagnosis and treatment. The practice has resulted in cutting back attending physicians' continued care of their hospitalized patients, in many instances reducing their teaching responsibilities which they carried jointly with staff physicians, as well as in their assignments to clinic services. It may also be affecting a continuum of care by the patient's primary physician. The impact of this trend is still to be determined. Where the practice has been in existence for some period, hospitals are seeking those departed "attendings" to return to serve the ambulatory primary and specialty clinics—which are the major sources of referral for the hospitalization of patients, thus filling beds. Their wish is to again have a continuing relationship to the institution.

Who will serve those vulnerable hospitalized patients in need? As short-stay hospitalizations have become the practice, it is likely that other personnel than social workers will become invested in discharge planning. Nurses or discharge aides will most likely assume that role. The aftercare needs of tertiary care patients will very likely fall to trained social workers in health care, initially in the institution and in community social agencies in liaison with the hospital's discharge planners.

While hospitals will seek to serve as the central overseer of the range of services identified, it is more likely that consortia and coalitions based in the community will have defined divisions of responsibility in order to implement specific aspects of service plans. Social workers will continue to function in community-based agencies, but will need to broaden their scope to offer social-health care, health-maintenance services, and specialized programs including health education.

Social workers will provide more social-health services to "at-home" patients who are known to private or agency-based physicians. "There is evidence of support for social work services as insurers, government and individuals" recognize their benefits and cost-effectiveness (Rehr and Rosenberg, 1991, p. 105). Even as reimbursement rates appear finite today, a number of capitation and managed care benefit plans have included a social work service formula. Also, social workers in hospitals have introduced services that, although still limited, include the private pay by clients, coverage by insurance, available social work care in physicians' group practice, and contracted plans between social agencies and government programs. In any of these arrangements of service, social work will need documentation to demonstrate the benefits of service. Demonstrating consumer and provider satisfaction with service will be a helpful evaluation tool (Rehr et al., 1998).

Whether hospital based or community agency based, social work will need to return to an earlier role by engaging in social epidemiological and survey methods in order to relate to their regional population's needs. In becoming more knowledgeable about local community residents, social workers can contribute to the institution and local agencies' recognition of social-health needs of individuals and families. They will translate those needs, wants, and findings in partnership with the community into program planning and implementation, lobbying jointly to seek support of projected plans, and enhancing the accountability of service providers to community residents, to regulators, and payers (Peake et al., 1998). Such studies will most likely be multiprofessional as social workers will join with other health care disciplines and with lay partners to address needs and to advocate for change and support.

There is already public advocacy for a shift from the primacy of provider-directed services to that of a patient-provider partnership. This should make care more patient-family related. While medical diagnosis and its treatment are central, social work will enhance both with the social assessment of patients and will join with other health care professionals to assist individuals and families with their physical and social functioning needs. Social work's emphasis on the family and the informal network makes it the most prepared health care profession to counsel an individual and his or her family so as to optimize lifestyle gains. Social workers will need to demonstrate that its services are cost-effective. Counseling will help to enhance the coping and motivational capacities of individuals. They will also be located in wellness and health maintenance programs tied in with physicians' care and will do early case-finding of persons at risk for illnesses. Early uncovering of persons with primary care needs would be referred to primary care physicians. In some ways, the interrelated social-health program proposed many years ago by the Kaiser Permanete Program (Garfield, 1970) could be depicted as shown in Figure 10.2.

Garfield's proposal (1970) projected a multitier system, separating the sick, early sick, worried well, and well. Each would enter a system of care and have access to what was needed in a comprehensive care program.

It is unlikely that social ailments such as person abuse and substance abuse will diminish in the immediate future. Such social problems cannot be left to medical care alone. In order to deal with the social disorders and with the introduction of prevention programs, social workers will join in task-organized teams to deal with the ailing and with advocacy for health education programs.

Social work has not made its services visible to the public and political entities. It will need to achieve recognition of its professional identity by its different constituents. As mentioned, the demonstration of the cost-benefits of its services becomes paramount in maintaining a key place in the delivery of social-health services. The private practice of social work will continue as the public is prepared to

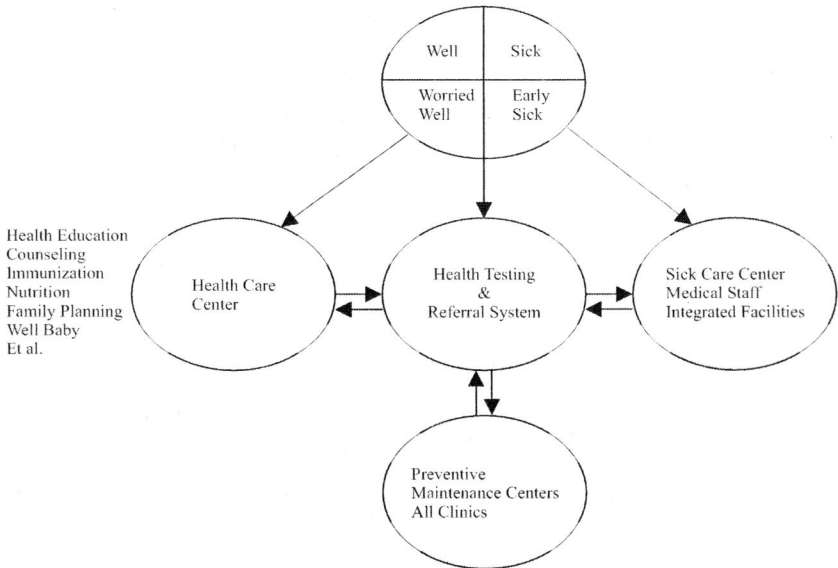

FIGURE 10.2. Proposed Social-Health Program

purchase counseling and support services for a range of social-health personal and family-related problems. Social workers provide the majority of psychosocial care today—more than psychologists and psychiatrists combined. Reimbursement plans will need to be negotiated with the different payer entities such as government, industry programs, and insurers. It is likely that there will be group capitation and managed care plans that will compensate for most referred social services. Social services could be provided by their own group practices, contractually related to covered plans and/or independently supported, or under company or corporate provision.

We agree with Pecukonis and colleagues (2003) that the changes in health care will have marked effects on the practice of social work. However, the outcome need not be negative. Much will depend on the field's leaders. Will they project the types of programs outlined? They will need to be not only service and program oriented but also social-health policy directed. Working with other health care providers would ensure a comprehensive social-health policy and the implementation of sound, affordable coverage for Americans. Collaboration with public partners will project both wants and needs to enhance the public health. Collaboration will remain the sine qua non of social work in health care (Rehr et al., 2000). Leadership does count. Rank and Hutchison (2000) defined leadership of social work as "the communication of vision, guided by the NASW Code of Ethics, to create proactive processes that empower individuals, families, groups, organizations and communities." They suggest "leadership is a process of advocacy and planning whereby an individual practices ethical and humanistic behavior to motivate others (clients and colleagues) to achieve common goals articulated by a shared vision" (p. 499). While leaders are not born, those who become leaders tend to demonstrate "vision," "goal-setting," "charisma," and "a personal capacity to inspire others" (Rosenberg and Katz, 2004).

Leadership skills and management capacities follow as learned characteristics that build on the personality characteristics described. The learning potential for leaders is also critical for practitioners. The academics and practitioners in social work have a responsibility to the field to create professionals who are knowledgeable, have enhanced skills, can collaborate with others (and with each other), can draw on studies to promote programs, remain accountable to those served and those who require services, and are committed to the "common good."

CONCLUSIONS

As authors of "Social Work and Health Care Yesterday, Today and Tomorrow," we projected a set of determinants and recommendations for the field of social work in health care—a field most meaningful to both of us based on our combined 100 years of practical, educational, administrative, and research experience. These multiple experiences in collaborative relationships in both medical and social work enterprises allowed us to project a set of conclusions that we reprise for social work deliberation:

> Make no mistake. Changes in health care have been dramatic and pivotal. Market forces are transforming the system, and how it is financed will affect what will be provided. Social work must be vigilant against the medicalization of its services. In the basic triad of public health (medicine, nursing, and social work), medical care remains significant for the sick, but health promotion becomes more meaningful. The most important determinants of health status are preventive services and quality-of-life standards.
>
> As the health system changes, social work in health care has three possible alternatives: decrying change and portraying it as diminishing in quality; sharing the plans of others for change; developing innovative programs in partnership with health care colleagues and the community. Evidence exists that social workers can take any one of the three pathways. However, creative social work leadership in partnership with creative social work staff can be the catalyst for innovation. Creative leadership will help support an informed public, particularly consumers of social work service, who will agree to and lobby for quality professional care. Professional social workers, particularly in academia, have always argued for a scientific base for practice, but this has been as difficult for social work to achieve as it has been for all behavioral sciences.
>
> The professional status of social work in health care is neither prescribed nor tidy. Just as the health care delivery system is

changing, so too must social work, for if it does not, it will have little reason to exist. Change should mean expanded roles: contributing to institutional status, resources, revenues, and programs while supporting access for prospective clients, eliminating fragmentation and obstacles to service, advocating for integration of care, counseling those in need, creating alliances in the community and with other medical institutions, for meeting social-health needs.

Social workers' experiences in clinical settings serve them as they observe client needs and recommend programs. They test the quality of service with the means available to them, in particular when they do applied studies and draw on their findings to enhance clinical knowledge and improve care. Collaboration is the sine qua non in health settings. The recognition that every health concern has a bio-psychosocial component has brought an interdisciplinary view of social-health care, which is attested to by an extensive partnership in practice.

Social workers have a curiosity about their practice that consists of live interactions, in which they seek to learn what is happening, why it is happening, and what will improve services. Observations prompt the questions that lead to exploration and ideas. As social workers "reflect-in-action," they move toward managing their professional selves and their relationships with others and toward a self-directed practice. The complexities of the health care institution and the autonomy of medical practice may well have served as models for social workers to seek their own autonomy and self-directedness. That sense of autonomy, combined with knowledge of the medical organization, has allowed them to advocate successfully on behalf of clients. The complexities of illness and disability have helped them value the tenet of family intercession and the meaning of ethical dilemmas and human values. This knowledge of the environment and community resources has informed individual client counseling and helped the institution recognize the need to share health care planning with local residents.

Competency and skill are governed by knowledge and experience. These are enhanced by professional accountability measures and by quality assurance. Social workers have learned to translate institutional missions and goals into services that benefit patients. Social workers also benefit the institution by providing early intervention and easier access to available resources for patients. Their services have had a value-added marketing effect for the institution and helped reduce the liability of risk.

Social work in the community has created better perceptions of providers and institutions among local residents. As social workers extend their boundaries beyond hospital walls, they see increased interest in their institutions in home care, nursing homes, long-term care, adult day care, schools, special housing, rehabilitation centers, assisted living care, primary care, and in wellness, prevention, and employee assistance programs. Social workers have applied health education in the direct client situation and in addressing the lay public.

With all that has been done to enhance the clinical enterprise, both in performance and in administration, social workers have assumed ongoing responsibility for their own continuing education, for educating tomorrow's social workers, and as key contributors to other health care professional education.

Much has been done, but so much lies ahead. These are critical times. How does social work safeguard its gains, thwart attacks on services, ensure professional survival, and promote programs into the next century? It must "come out of the closet," so to speak. It must be visible, market its services, educate its constituencies, participate in policy deliberation, and, above all, demonstrate the benefits of service to individuals and their families, the communities and its providers, and those who regulate and pay for care.

Beyond its commitment to the profession, social work must join in coalitions with other health care professions and the public, to secure and support providing human service. As medical care institutions and providers negotiate with insurers and other payers, commitment to the uninsured and underinsured must enter into the deliberations. As downsizing continues, where will further cuts be made? Safeguarding quality and access must be paramount in commitment to the public. Social work education must move beyond its academic walls and enter into academic-practice partnership with public health professionals, the people, and the business community. Joint planning will help social workers face today's social-health problems, the changing environment, the fiscal crisis, the reengineering of health care delivery, and will determine the realities of social work practice for today and tomorrow.*

A social-health policy based on people-related needs rather than on provider service provisions is a national health program essential. Provision for care that guarantees access to all and is equitable, affordable, available, financially sound, fair to providers, and ensures ongoing assessment for quality and accountability is a public health policy requirement.

Source: "Social Work and Health Care: Yesterday, Today and Tomorrow" by H. Rehr and G. Rosenberg (Ch. 5, pp. 86-122). From *Social Work at the Millennium,* edited by June Gary Hopps and Robert Morris. Copyright © 2000 by June Gary Hopps and Robert Morris. Reprinted with permission of The Free Press, a Division of Simon & Schuster Adult Publishing Group. All rights reserved.

Appendix I

Directors, Department of Social Work Service

1906-1907	Jennie Greenthal, RN, Chief; replaced by a nurse, name unknown.
1908-1915	Rose L. Johnson, RN, Headworker; left to become the Superintendent of the Solomon and Betty Loeb Home. An assistant worker was hired in 1909 due to the growing workload.
1916	Evelyn Troumbley, RN, Headworker.
1917-1921	Mrs. Mabel Montgomery Boorum, RN, Headworker; left to become the Executive Director, Hospital Social Services Association. During the war, four nurse social workers left with the Mount Sinai Unit, Base Hospital No. 3.
1921-1923	Ida Fishkin, AB, Headworker.
5/1/23-8/53	Fanny Lissauer G. Mendelsohn, BS, RN (MSH School of Nursing, 1913), Headworker (title changed to Director 1925). Due to work load, an assistant Headworker was appointed, Mary Hallahan.
9/53-1970	Doris Siegel, MS, Director appointed, following a study of the social work services to professionalize the department. Associate Director Helen Rehr was appointed in 1954.
1970-1971	Helen Rehr, DSW/PhD, Acting Director.
1971-1981	Helen Rehr, DSW/PhD, Director; Janice Paneth, MSW, and Gary Rosenberg, PhD, Associate Directors.
1981-1986	Gary Rosenberg, PhD, Director; Andrew Weissman, PhD, Associate Director.
1986-1988	Andrew Weissman, PhD, Director.
1988-Present	Susan Blumenfield, DSW, Director; Susan Bernstein, DSW, Associate Director.

Appendix II

Edith J. Baerwald Professors of Community Medicine (Social Work) and Chairpersons, Division of Social Work and Behavioral Sciences

1965-1970   Doris Siegel, MS
1971-1986   Helen Rehr, DSW/PhD
1986-Present Gary Rosenberg, PhD

Appendix III

Chairpersons, Auxiliary Board

Term	Names
1916-1917	Edith Lehman (Mrs. Herbert H. Lehman)
1917-1949	Ruth Cook (Mrs. Alfred A. Cook)
1949-1956	Hortense Hirsch (Mrs. Walter A. Hirsch)
1956-1961	Helen Benjamin (Mrs. Robert M. Benjamin)
1961-1966	Henrietta Weil (Mrs. Frank L. Weil)
1966-1971	Jane Aron (Mrs. Jack R. Aron)
1971-1976	Ruth Klein (Mrs. Seymour Klein)
1976-1981	Mary C. Wolf (Mrs. Stephen L. Wolf)
1981-1986	Patricia S. Levinson (Mrs. Robert A. Levinson)
1986-1991	Edith Schur (Mrs. Marvin H. Schur)
1991-1996	Karen H. Freedberg (Mrs. David S. Freedberg)
1996-2000	Jean C. Crystal (Mrs. James W. Crystal)
2000-Present	Sue K. Feld (Mrs. Stuart P. Feld)

Appendix IV

Social Work Events

1925

Board of Trustees determines that social work records should be added to the regular history of the patient.

1927

Social workers assigned to services (medical and surgical) rather than to the wards.
Jewish Social Services Association (JSSA) doing work on mental health wards.
Special course for social workers funded.

1928

Salary differential between psychiatric and staff workers.
Social workers to receive name plates.

1930

Educator for staff employed from Cook Fund.
Case meetings begun.

1933

First two social work students from New York University in placement at Mount Sinai five hours per week.

1937

Two students from Teachers College.

1941

Discussion of social work role in war.

1952

Committee to work with Mrs. Moss from Auxiliary, Medical Board, and Administration.
Social work to be assigned to follow up Jewish patients discharged from Bellevue.

1957

Board investigated staffing at Saint Vincent's Hospital Psychiatric Services.

1959

Letter to NASW regarding professional responsibility.

1962

Special research fund established in November.

1963

Budgets of Auxiliary Board and Social Service separated.

1964

Social work salaries in line with Federation agencies.

1965

Gave two full scholarships for social work degrees with two-year commitment.

1966

For ten years Auxiliary had given money for two college students to work as case aides for eight weeks in summer; in 1966 approved two more from Southern Negro colleges.

1967

Funded researcher for Social Health Advocate Program.

1969

Edith J. Baerwald Professor of Community Medicine (social work) is established at the Mount Sinai Medical School.

Mr. Joseph Klingenstein gave special grant to study how social work can contribute to medical education.

1971

Gift from Mrs. Benjamin for conjoint medical and social work education experience for students in the health professions.

1972

Membership established for the Doris Siegel Memorial Committee.

1973

Consortium with Hunter started.

1974

Medicine and Social Work, edited by Helen Rehr, is published by Prodist Press.

Board established Baerwald discretionary fund.

1975

Dr. Regensburg's study is published by Harper & Row: *Toward Education for the Health Professions.*

1978

Ethical Dilemmas in Health Care, edited by Helen Rehr, is published by Prodist Press.

1979

Professional Accountability for Social Work Practice, edited by Helen Rehr, is published by Prodist Press.

1981

In the Patients' Interest, edited by Mildred Mailick and Helen Rehr, is published by Prodist Press.

1982

Milestones in Social Work and Medicine, edited by Helen Rehr, is published by Prodist Press.

1983

Advancing Social Work Practice in the Health Care Field, edited by Gary Rosenberg and Helen Rehr, is published by The Haworth Press.
Social Work Issues in Health Care, edited by Rosalind S. Miller and Helen Rehr, is published by Prentice-Hall.

1986

A New Model in Academic-Practice Partnership: Multi-Instructor and Institutional Collaboration in Social Work, edited by Helen Rehr and Phyllis Caroff, is published by Ginn Press.

1988

Social Work in Health Care Management: The Move to Leadership, edited by Gary Rosenberg and Sylvia Clarke, is published by The Haworth Press.

1991

The Changing Context of Social Health Care, edited by Helen Rehr and Gary Rosenberg, is published by The Haworth Press.

1994

Social Work in Ambulatory Care, edited by Gary Rosenberg and Andrew Weissman, is published by The Haworth Press.

1998

Creative Social Work in Health Care, edited by Helen Rehr, Gary Rosenberg, and Susan Blumenfeld, is published by the Springer Press.

2000

Behavioral Social Work in Health Care Settings, edited by Gary Rosenberg and Andrew Weissman, is published by The Haworth Press.

2001

Clinical Data-Mining in Practice-Based Research: Social Work in Hospital Settings, edited by Irwin Epstein and Susan Blumenfield, is published by The Haworth Press.

2005

Clinical and Research Uses of an Adolescent Mental Health Intake Questionnaire, edited by Ken Peake, Irwin Epstein, and Daniel Medeiros, is published by the Haworth Press.

Appendix V

Auxiliary Board Projects, 1969 to 2004

Project Name	Year
Inquiry into Social Work Practice in Hospitals	1969
Play Program—Pediatrics and Obstetrics Clinics	1972
Patients' Benefit Survey	1973
Screening Children of East Harlem for Speech and Hearing Disorders	1975
Breast Models for Instruction in Self-Examination	1976
Termination of Green Box	1976
Patient Activity Program	1976
Spanish Interpreter (for period between funding)	1976
Diabetic ID Tags	1977
Air Conditioning (a part of Gift Shop renovation)	1977
Cooperative Apartments	1977
Study of Patient Representative Programs in the United States	1977
Development of Employee Assistance Program	1978
Hospitality Program	1978
Social Work Planning Model	1978
After-School Tutorial	1978
Legislative Committee Grant	1978
Social Work Services Legislative Grant	1978
CPR Instruction for Members of the Community	1978
Social Work–Psychiatry Collaboration for Medicaid Reimbursement	1979
Gift Shop Public Relations Grant	1979
Visitors Guide	1979
Clinical Management of Diabetes—Demonstration Project	1979
Imagination Workshop	1979
Saf-T-Pops	1979
Pediatric Play Therapy Program—Inpatient Unit	1980

Project Name	Year
Densitometer	1980
The Mount Sinai Volunteer Newsletter (start-up money)	1980
Ventilating System—Gift Shop Storeroom	1980
Hemophilia Clinic Project	1980
Legislative Round Table—Home Health Care	1980
Pediatric Acute Care—Holding Area of Emergency Room TV Cameras	1980
Restoration of Portrait of Meyer Guggenheim	1980
Casebook on Epidemiology for Social Workers	1981
Patient Representative Program Study	1981
Operating Room Family Waiting Room	1082
Health Education Center Coordinator	1983
TV Sets for Day Rooms—Guggenheim 2 and Housman 1	1983
Center for the Study of Women's Health—A Feasibility Study	1983
Legislative Aides Day	1983
Juvenile Diabetes Teaching Service	1984
Pain Management Service	1984
Child Life Specialist	1985
Telephone Outreach	1985
Marketing of Communicard	1986
Enhancement of Employment Status Following Coronary Bypass Surgery	1986
Support of Archivist for Medical Center	1986
Volunteer Department Refurbishing	1986
Improving Physicians' Communication Skills	1987
Beautician Services	1987
Pediatric Calorimetry Program	1987
East Harlem Adolescent Project	1988
Dean's Continuing Medical Education Seminars	1988
R.E.A.P—Entitlement Program	1988
Geriatric Evaluation and Treatment Unit	1988
Patients' Library Book Return Project	1988
Health Education Translation Project	1988
Pediatric Development Evaluation Service	1988
Pediatric Clinic Child Life Program	1989
Nurse Recruitment Program	1989
M.O.M.S.—Peer Mentor Project for Teens	1989
Young Professionals Volunteer Program	1989
Pediatric School-Based Health Project	1990

Project Name	Year
Parent Sharing—Neonatal Intensive Care Unit	1990
Cost of Care for Pediatric AIDS	1990
R.E.A.P. Automation Project	1990
Discharge Follow-Up Study—Service Component	1990
Bioethics Consortium Colloquium	1991
Early Child Health Project	1991
Mount Sinai Comprehensive Breast Cancer Service	1991
From Home to Hospital—Easing the Transition	1991
Holocaust Survivors' Project	1991
Nurse Physician Collaboration for Quality Patient Care	1992
Patient Library Metal Book Carts	1992
Proxy Distribution and Continuing Patient Care Project	1992
Audio Visual Film for Hearing Impaired	1992
Menopause Group Services in the Community	1992
Star Theater Project—Interactive Project for Teens	1992
Pediatric Patients' Procedures Library Project	1993
Social Work Liaison Project—AIDS Volunteers	1993
Stroke Club Project	1993
Infant Car Seat Program	1993
Childhood Cancer Resource Program	1993
Mount Sinai Student Community Volunteer Opportunities Project	1993
Spinal Cord Social Work Project	1993
Continuous Quality Improvement Initiative	1994
Parent Educator Project	1994
Mount Sinai Little Sisters Collaborative Early Intervention Project	1994
Hotel Accommodations Coordinator Position	1994
Physician Partnership Project	1994
Patient Library Automation Project	1995
Palliative Care Project	1995
Walking Tall	1995
Parents And Children Together (PACT)	1995
Alzheimer's Disease Respite Care, Support and Training Program	1996
Doing It Right—Wellness for the Larger Woman	1996
Enhanced Asthma Management for Inner-City Children	1996
Domestic Violence Prevention and Education	1996
Improving Care for Patients with Congestive Heart Failure	1996

Project Name	Year
Project Linkage—Social Work Services Coordinator	1996
Lead and the Origins of Urban Youth Violence	1997
Healthy Families, Healthy Lives	1997
COSTEP (Community Stroke Education Program)	1997
Book Boxes for Patients' Library	1997
Adult Diabetic Patient Education Program Evaluation	1998
Reach Out and Read	1998
A Lending Library for NICU Patients	1998
Mount Sinai Specialty Unit in Environmental Pediatrics	1998
Face to Face	1999
Assisting Our Patients to Surf into the 21st Century	1999
Orthodox Services Project	1999
Reaching the Neediest of the Needy	1999
Child Health Insurance Outreach	1999
Family Violence Prevention Risk Identification and Early Intervention	2000
Family Resource Center Library—Maternal and Child Health Center	2000
Educational Program for CAPP Caregiver	2000
Young Fathers Program—Renewal	2001
MOMS Summer Employment Program	2001
Pet-Assisted Therapy Program	2001
Health Promotion Services for Older Adults	2002
Development of an Acute Musculoskeletal Medicine Clinic	2002
The GYN Patient Support Program	2003
Nurse Practitioner Coordinator for GI Clinic	2004
Pediatric Dental Clinic Enhancement	2004

Appendix VI

Women As Volunteers

Helen Rehr, DSW

INTRODUCTION

The women associated with The Mount Sinai Hospital have given service to patients, their families, and the community from the hospital's beginning in 1852. Their early recognition that many patients were vulnerable and required more than medical care led them to volunteer their services. In the early days, they volunteered themselves or their domestic staff to assist with essential tasks of the hospital. They provided needed materials as well. In addition, they assisted those sick vulnerable women and men who could leave the hospital to return to their community with needed welfare.

As times changed and awareness of the social and environmental impact on the public welfare grew, women organized in the community to relieve the worst conditions by charitable acts (Morris, 2000, p. 43),* and those of the hospital organized within. The Social Service Auxiliary was created in 1917 to provide assistance to the vulnerable sick. Its primary purpose was to promote the general welfare of the patient and family and thus to enhance patient care. The number of volunteer women grew, developing and broadening the original mission with the result of bringing social services, special programs, and amenities to hospital patient care. They became advocates for improvement of social-health conditions in the community. They also contributed to the enhancement of the education of health care professionals and encouraged the study of social-health issues to improve care (see Chapter 3).

The personal history of an Auxiliary Board member, which follows, reflects the evolving experience of a woman volunteer from her beginning at the hospital to a later stage of leadership and becoming a member of the

---

*Morris, R. (2000). "Social Work's Century of Evaluation As a Profession." In *Social Work at the Millennium,* edited by J. G. Hopps and R. Morris. New York: Free Press, p. 43.

hospital's Board of Trustees. Mrs. Walter A. Hirsch presents her experience as an Auxiliary Board member (Hirsch, W.A., personal history of auxillary board member, Mount Sinai Archives, unpublished).

A PERSONAL HISTORY OF AN AUXILIARY BOARD MEMBER

Having been a volunteer since 1917, I have seen a great change take place. At first, we volunteers were considered Lady Bountifuls, patronizing, and we certainly were not popular—sort of a drug on the market—to be tolerated and suffered.

Then during the First World War, suddenly we had our opportunity. We were needed due to shortages and difficulties in getting personnel.

It was at that time that I took the Red Cross Social Service course, passed my examination, and then appeared for my first assignment. My supervisor took one look at me, and decided then and there that I was no good, so she assigned me to the most difficult and unpleasant case in the district. I went to a tenement on the Upper West Side, to an Italian family with two sons in the service. The husband was a barber, and there were five or six children at home. There was a newborn, sickly, lying naked on the bed. The place was dirty, smelly; there was no equipment, nor were there any toilet facilities. I took the sick baby, wrapped in a filthy shawl, in a taxi to the Vanderbilt Clinic, and waited around for the doctor and the diagnosis. Finally the diagnosis was given me: the baby was a congenital syphilitic. I was scared to death but determined to carry on. I took the infant home, and returned to the Red Cross, wrote up the case, turned it in, and waited. The supervisor sent for me and said: "Mrs. Hirsch, I never thought you would stick it out." Some time later I told her that she had almost ruined my social service career.

It is a far cry from that scene to being a Volunteer today.

The development in medical social service in every branch of philanthropic endeavor has proven that we are a serious group of workers just as intent on the job as the paid professional.

And now to Mount Sinai where I have worked for 29 years.

- Did you know that the Mount Sinai and Bellevue Social Service departments were started in 1906, a year after Dr. Richard Cabot started this first experiment at the Massachusetts General Hospital in Boston?
- Then in 1916 the Social Service Auxiliary was formed by women volunteers "to attend to the many wants of convalescent patients and the patient's family."

- Mrs. Herbert Lehman was our first President, and when she went to Washington, because of her husband's duties in the First World War, Mrs. Alfred Cook succeeded her, and remained the President for 34 years. I became a member of the Social Service Auxiliary in 1923.

I am going to give you a few dates that may be of interest in showing the development of Social Service.

- In 1919 the Children's Health Class was formed. This Class was the forerunner of our child-parent clinic, in other words, our Children's Psychiatric Department of today. It was in this Children's Health Class that I had my first volunteer job at Mount Sinai.
- In 1924 the Occupational Therapy Department was started at Mount Sinai in the Social Service Department.
- In 1933 our Rehabilitation workroom was established—I think the first of its kind in the country, and it is still a unique activity of our Social Service and an example of work of this Department.

B.B., who was born in Poland, had an accident to her eyes as a child. This necessitated the removal of the left eye, which was followed by a serious infection, causing a good deal of destruction of facial tissue. B.B. was badly disfigured when she arrived in this country. Her family finally brought her to our hospital for treatment. She was admitted for cosmetic surgery and numerous operations were performed over a period of 10 years. As a result of this and the fact that she had no normal activities, she became withdrawn, unsure of herself, shy and unhappy, and she had no hope for the future. About six years ago she was admitted to our Workroom, which she attended regularly between hospitalizations and periods of convalescent care. Gradually her reluctance to mingle with people and her shyness disappeared. The Workroom experience helped her to overcome many feelings of inferiority and in her own words, "it saved my life." It showed her that she was capable of producing something useful and that she had even more than average skills. Her facial restoration was quite successful, and with the help of her confidence gained in the Workroom and with social service support, it was possible to refer her to the State Department of Vocational Rehabilitation where she received specialized training. B.B. has now been employed full time in a manufacturing plant for several months. Her entire personality has changed. She is cheerful, more independent and confident of her ability to handle herself. Out of a group of 30 people, six were rehabilitated to the extent that they are now back in the real commercial, competitive world.

Each year we open a shop, The Green Box, for several months before the holiday season, where articles made by people in the Workroom are sold.

Many of you have perhaps patronized this shop and know what really excellent work is done.

We have the following setup at Mount Sinai: 1) a Social Service Auxiliary, given new name (the prior one is a misnomer), because under the Social Service Auxiliary we include all our women's activities. We are in the process of looking for a better name, such as Women's Division, or Women's Social Service Committee, and 2) a Volunteer Department.

While the two are closely related, they are two separate volunteer departments within the hospital.

First, I would like to tell you about the Social Service Auxiliary. In 1949 our by-laws were revised, and the objectives changed to the following: a) to supplement the medical care provided by the hospital by such service as will further the welfare of the patient and his family, and b) to render such other service to the hospital as may from time to time be approved by the Board of Trustees of the Hospital.

The Auxiliary is composed of 30 Board members. All members are elected by our own Board. A new member must be proposed by the Nominating Committee which has looked into her background. She is chosen for various reasons, such as experience and interest in community affairs, from the group of Volunteers, or for such other reasons as would seem to make her a valuable member of the group.

Above all, the Board member should have her role in the agency made clear to her when she is asked to serve. She should not consider herself a figurehead, nor an expert.

The activities which the Social Service Auxiliary are concerned with are financed by funds which are partly secured from the Federation of Jewish Philanthropies, and from the United Hospital Fund by yearly grants. Insofar as these do not cover the expenses of the Auxiliary Board's activities, the remainder is considered an operational expense by the Hospital and is paid out of operational funds.

The Social Service Auxiliary also enjoys some funds which have been built up over the years through its own contributions, or contributions secured by its members. These funds are used to pay for non-budgetary items, experimental work such as scholarships to social workers to finish their education, or expenses toward day camp for children known to the Hospital. They may be used for any and every purpose by the Auxiliary at its discretion, except those funds which are, or were contributed for special purposes, and such allocations are of course respected.

As we do not solicit funds, I think every Board member of a Federation agency owes financial allegiance to the Federation.

Before assuming any responsibility, a new Board member must know her hospital thoroughly; must learn what our responsibilities are as members of the Social Service Auxiliary within the framework of the overall hospital picture.

After this orientation, every member must accept the responsibility of either heading one of the sub-committees, or of serving on one of the committees, such as the following: Social Service Committee, Recreation Education, Scholarship, Gift Shop, Workroom, Library, Occupational Therapy, Public Relations, Maternity, and many others. The newest is the Recreation Committee. Naturally in these assignments we consider the abilities and special interest of the members and place them where they can be the happiest and most valuable.

To digress for a moment, my experience with the Gift Shop started in 1933, when I became a Trustee of Mount Sinai. At that time I made a thorough survey of the Gift Shop situation in other hospitals and the report of my findings was the first report that I had ever made before the august body of Trustees. As I left for the Trustee meeting, my husband said, "I hope your sense of humor will not interfere with the acceptance of your report." So I went up to the meeting not too happy, and very insecure. When I got on my feet, I was trembling like a leaf and gave my report in a halting voice. A motion to accept the report was made by President George Blumenthal and I waited with bated breath to find that it was unanimously *not* accepted. To say the least, I was frustrated, because as I was leaving, every Trustee came up to me and told me it was a good report, but each one had turned me down.

Now I am glad to say that the attitude has changed, and our Gift Shop is a great asset. It started last summer and is booming.

An important function of our Board members is to come to the Case Committee meetings which take place twice a month, where the staff and Board members meet to hear about, and discuss important and difficult cases. At these meetings, the professional and lay people meet on a shared participating level.

The amount of time that members of the Auxiliary give to the work varies. If there is a special job to be done, I have known a member to come to the Hospital daily, but that is not the usual procedure. However, we are always on call.

Due to the fact that we are 36 years old, we are having a professional make a reevaluation and reappraisal of our activities. We want to be sure that we are functioning with the highest efficiency and that we are including only those activities which properly come within the scope of the Social Service Auxiliary.

As an example, we now know, as the result of a survey made by the co-chairpersons of our Volunteer Department, that the Volunteer Department should not be a part of the Social Service Auxiliary, but should be a separate department of the Hospital, with the same status as the Social Service Auxiliary. After all, volunteers comprise a group that is just as distinct and individual as any other group within the Hospital. Therefore this Volunteer Department should be directly responsible to the Hospital Administrator, operating under a professional Director of Volunteers. The new Volunteer Department is now functioning as a separate department with a full-time professional administrator. At the last census, we had 170 volunteers who gave 3,686 hours of service during a one-month period.

To quote from this survey: "The need for volunteers is increasing with the expansion of the medical, surgical, and psychiatric services, and with the shortages, the big turnover of nurses, social service workers, and hospital personnel. This necessitates constant fresh ideas for recruitment, and close cooperation with the director of personnel of the Hospital."

This survey included a study of the Volunteer Department in the voluntary hospitals which most closely resembled Mount Sinai, namely New York Hospital, Lenox Hill, Presbyterian, St. Luke's, Roosevelt, Beth Israel and Montefiore. While differences in organizational structure existed among all of them, they each had a professional head of the Volunteer Department.

We also found that volunteers must be provided with proper headquarters, including a lounge, adequate washing up and toilet facilities, lockers, filing equipment, and a private office for the Director of Volunteers, etc., etc.

We know that volunteers are a means of improving public relations. A satisfied volunteer spreads good feelings and enlarges the Hospital's circle of friends. A dissatisfied volunteer can do the Hospital irreparable harm.

It stands to reason that the core of a successful Volunteer Department must be in the initial interviewing and placement. Strict requirements, such as medical references, as well as social references, which are demanded of the paid personnel should also be required from the volunteer and carefully considered before acceptance of the volunteer. Also, a minimum number of hours of service per week should be required on the application form. Volunteers in a modern hospital must realize that they are a part of a team of professional and lay workers, and that placement, training, and supervision by a professional are essential to such a program.

It is important that the policies of the Hospital be thoroughly interpreted to the volunteer and that she know what part she is expected to play in the overall hospital picture. Proper orientation of a volunteer is a means of attaining better work.

It has been estimated that it takes fifteen hours of a paid worker's time to train a new volunteer.

Perhaps you will be surprised to know that there is a definite monetary saving to the Hospital in terms of the cost of paid personnel. On the basis of the minimum wage scale of $.75 per hour, 1,000 hours of volunteer service would be estimated at a savings of $750.

Please remember, however, that volunteers should only be placed in positions where funds are not allocated for paid personnel. *Volunteers supplement the paid personnel.* They do not replace them.

You are probably wondering how we recruit volunteers. Most of our volunteers are self-referred. We get them from schools and colleges during vacation time. We secure them from the United Hospital Fund Volunteer Service, through doctors, through other volunteers, through the Red Cross, from churches, synagogues, temples, clubs, high schools and junior high schools and College Placement Bureaus and of course through Federation.

At this point, I would like to say a word about this volunteer course which you are all taking. To me, it has been one of the most outstanding programs in which Federation has ever engaged. You who are here today are proof of that for you are actually preparing for your roles as volunteers in many fields.

One of the most important things to consider is the interviewing of a volunteer. I quote from an article in the July 1951 issue of *HIGHLIGHTS,* called "Interviewing in a Volunteer Bureau":

"One must make the first contact with the Volunteer Bureau a positive experience for the individual who has expressed interest in welfare work."

"The volunteer must understand too, that her loyalty and responsibility will belong to the agency of which she becomes, by nature of her services, a non-paid staff member."

In order to do effective volunteer work in a hospital, there is need for a flexible, adaptable personality as from time to time hospitals must shift volunteers around.

Many times it has been found that a volunteer comes with a special job in mind for which she is not fitted. In placements this fact must be duly recognized and this requires tact and understanding on both sides. There should be continuous reviewing of job opportunities.

At Mount Sinai, volunteers are assigned to work as follows:

Information Desk	Receptionist
Hospital Admitting Room	Secretarial—clerical work
Hospital Record Room	Secretarial—clerical work
OPD Admitting Physician	Clerical
OPD Clinics	Receptionist (and special assignments)
Patients' Library	Taking books, magazines, cards and games to the wards on a cart.
Research Library	Stenographic and clerical assistance to librarian.
Kindergarten	Assist Kindergartner with individual and group recreation.

Ward Rounds	Assist Chief of Service with special work. Clerical and getting information for research.
Research Work	Assigned to assist doctors with special projects. Sending out follow-up letters, etc.
Surgical Clinics	Red Cross Nurses' Aides—assist with dressing and with sterilizing instruments, etc.
Blood Bank	Registrar—and assisting donors.
Wards	Red Cross Nurses' Aides—assist nurses.
Wards	Other volunteers to assist with clerical work. Diet slips, etc. Also answer telephone.
Occupational Therapy	Volunteers who have had a course in O.T. assist regular staff.
Laboratories	Washing glassware, etc.
X-ray Department	Assist with patients.
Maternity	Baby Alumni Fund—providing layettes.
Recreation	Newest Project—assist with activities.

A pilot experiment in Recreation was tried out this past Fall in Ward K at Mount Sinai Hospital. This is the first time this has ever been attempted in a general acute care voluntary hospital.

Mrs. Beatrice Hill, Recreation Consultant to the Rehabilitation Service of Bellevue Hospital and the Goldwater Memorial Hospital, and the Institute of Physical Medicine and Rehabilitation, volunteered her time and that of several assistants for this project. This experiment proved so successful that we are now trying out a Recreation program throughout the Hospital wards for one year.

Volunteers are playing a most important role in providing this Recreation program. Working girls are volunteers in the evening. That is the low ebb period for patients in the hospital.

I have tried to be specific today, and hope that when I have finished, you will feel free to ask me questions which may bring out certain aspects of this most important part of hospital work, that in my allotted time I have been unable to cover.

To me the rewards of Volunteer Service are the personal satisfaction we get from rendering help wherever we are needed; the gratification we derive from a job well done; and the realization that we are part of a team of people who are trying to better the health of the individuals who make up the community in which we live.

To quote from the New York Times of May 11, 1952, "Through the unselfish efforts of volunteers, the care and comfort of millions of hospital patients are being enhanced, and the service of hospitals widened and strengthened."

Mrs. Walter A. Hirsch
Submitted June 1952

References

Chapter 1

Kerson, T. S. (1981). *Medical Social Work, the Pre-Professional Paradox*. New York: Irvington Publication.

Lyons, A. S. and Petrucelli, R. J. (1978). *Medicine: An Illustrated History*. New York: Harry W. Abrams, Inc.

Chapter 2

Bosch, S. J. and Deuschle, K. D. (1989). "Social Work: An Important Component of Community Medicine at Mount Sinai School of Medicine." *The Mount Sinai Journal of Medicine,* 56(6), pp. 459-467.

Cahill, T. (1999). *The Gift of the Jews: How a Tribe of Desert Nomads Changed the Way Everyone Thinks and Feels*. New York: Anchor Books.

Cannon, I. M. (1952). *On the Social Fronts of Medicine*. Boston: Harvard University Press.

Lyons, A. S. and Petrucelli, R. J. (1978). *An Illustrated History*. New York: Harry W. Abrams, Inc.

MacKenzie, R. (1919). "Medical Social Service and the Hospital Organization." *Hospital Social Service, 1*(2), p. 95.

Rehr, H. and Rosenberg, G. (2002)."Social Work and Health Care, Yesterday, Today and Tomorrow." In *Social Work at the Millennium,* J. G. Hopps and R. Morris (eds.). New York: Free Press.

Thomas, L. (1981). "Therapy." *Atlantic Monthly,* April, p. 42.

Chapter 3

Axinn, J. and Levin, H. (1975). *A History of the American Response to Need*. New York: Harper and Row.

Cannon, I. M. (1933). "The Function of Medical Social Services in the United States." *Hospital Social Services,* XXVII (1), January, pp. 1-16.

Cannon, I. M. (1952). *On the Social Fronts of Medicine*. Boston: Harvard University Press.

Cassell, E. J. (1986). "Ideals in Conflict." *Daedalus,* Spring.

Cluff, L. E. (1986). "America's Romance with Medicine and Medical Science." *Daedalus*, Spring, p. 153.

Deutsch, (1946). A. *The Mentally Ill in the United States*. New York: Columbia University Press.

Dodds, T. M. (1993). "Richard Cabot Medical Reformer During the Progressive Era." *Annals of Internal Medicine*, 119 (5), pp. 417-422.

Ebert, R. H. (1973). "The Medical School." *Life and Death and Medicine—A Scientific American Book* (p. 84). San Francisco: W. H. Freeman.

Flexner, A. (1915). "Is Social Work a Profession?" National Conference of Charities and Corrections Proceedings 42, Baltimore, Maryland, May 12-19, p. 587.

Johnson, K. (1986). "Reaching Out to the Community." *Daedalus*, Spring, p. 163.

Knowles, J. H. (1973). "The Hospital." *Life and Death of Medicine—A Scientific American Book*. San Francisco: W. H. Freeman.

Leiby, J. (1978). *A History of Social Welfare and Social Work in the United States*. New York: Columbia University Press.

Lowe, J. and Herranen, M. (1978). "Conflict in Teamwork: Understanding Roles and Relationships." *Social Work in Health Care*, 3 (3).

Lowe, J. and Herranen, M. (1981). "Understanding Teamwork: And the Look at the Concepts." *Social Work in Health Care*, 7 (1).

Lyons, A. S. and Petrucelli, R. J. (1978). *Medicine, An Illustrated History*. New York: Harry N. Abrams, Inc.

MacEachern, M. T. (1940). *Hospital Organization Management*. Chicago: Physician Record Co., pp. 109-112.

Rehr, H. (ed.) (1982). *Milestones in Social Work and Medicine*. New York: Prodist.

Rehr, H. and Rosenberg, G. (2000). "Social Work in Health Care: Today and Tomorrow." In *Social Work at the Millennium*, J. G. Hopps and R. Morris (eds.) (pp. 86-122). New York: The Free Press.

Richmond, M. (1917). *Social Diagnosis*. New York: Russell Sage Foundation.

Rogers, D. (1986). "The Early Years." *Daedalus*, Spring, pp. 1-18.

Rosenberg, C. (1967). "The Practice of Medicine in New York City a Century Ago." *Bulletin of the History of Medicine*, 41, May-June, pp. 223-224.

Rosenberg, G. and Clarke, S. (1987). *Social Workers in Health Care Management: The Move to Leadership*. New York: The Haworth Press.

Rosner, D. K. (1978). "A Once Charitable Enterprise." Doctoral dissertation, Harvard University, Cambridge Massachusetts. May.

Starr, P. (1980). *The Transformation of American Medicine*. New York: Basic Books.

Stein, Florence (1953). "The Social Service Department of the Mount Sinai Hospital—A History: A Report to the Mount Sinai Auxilliary Board." Mimeograph.

Williams, T. F. (1950). "Cabot, Peabody, and the Care of the Patient." *Bulletin of the History of Medical Allied Science*, 24, pp. 462-481.

Chapter 4

Austin, D. (2000). "The Second Century: A Forward Look from a Historical Prespective." In *Social Work at the Millennium,* J. G. Hopps and R. Morris (eds.). New York: Free Press, pp. 18-41.
Axinn, J. and Levin, H. (1995). *Social Welfare: A History of the American Response to Need.* New York: Harper and Row, p. 44.
Cannon, I. M. (1952). *On the Social Frontier of Medicine.* Boston: Harvard University Press.
Caroff, P. and Rehr, H. (eds.) (1985). *A New Model in an Academic-Practice Partnership.* Lexington, MA: Ginn Press.
Hirsch, J. and Doherty, B. (1952). *The First Hundred Years of Mount Sinai of New York, 1852-1952.* New York: Random House, pp. 14-15, 151.
Knowles, J. H. (1973). "The Hospital." In *Life and Death of Medicine—A Scientific American Book.* San Francisco: W. H. Freeman, p. 92.
MacEachern, M. T. (1940). *Hospital Organizational Management.* Chicago: Physicians Record Co.
Regensberg, J. (1979). *Toward Education for Health Professions.* New York: Harper and Row.
Rehr, H. (ed.) (1982). *Milestones in Social Work and Medicine.* New York: Prodist.
Rosenberg, C. (1967). "The Practice of Medicine in New York a Century Ago." *Bulletin of the History of Medicine,* 41, May-June.
Rosner, D. K. (1978). *A Once Charitable Enterprise.* Doctoral dissertation, Harvard University, Cambridge, Massachusetts. May.
Snyder, C. (2004). "Radical Civic Virtue: Women in the 19th Century Civil Society." *New Political Science,* 26 (1), pp. 51-69.
Starr, P. (1982). *The Transformation of American Medicine.* New York: Basic Books, p. 155.
Stein, F. T. (1953). "The Social Service Department of the Mount Sinai Hospital—A History." Mimeograph.

Chapter 5

Aufses, A. H. Jr. and Niss, B. I. (2002). *The House of Noble Deeds: The Mount Sinai Hospital, 1852-2002.* New York: University Press.
Berkman, B. and Rehr, H. (1966). "A Study of Aging Ward Patients Served." The Mount Sinai Medical Center, June. Unpublished monograph.
Epstein, I. and Blumenfield, S. (2001). *Clinical Data-Mining in Practice-Based Research in Hospital Settings.* Binghamton, NY: The Haworth Press.
Rehr, H. (1979). *Professional Accountability for Social Work Practice.* New York: Neale Watson Academic Publishing.

Rehr, H. and Caroff, P. (1986). *A New Model in Academic-Practice Partnership: Multi-Instructor and Institutional Collaboration in Social Work.* Lexington, MA: Ginn Press.

Rehr, H., Rosenberg, G., and Blumenfield, S. (1998). *Creative Social Work in Health Care.* New York: Springer Publishing Co.

Sweet, A. and White, E. (1961). "Social and Functional Rehabilitation of Patients with Severe Poliomyelitis." *The Mount Sinai Journal of Medicine,* 28.

Chapter 7

Berkman, B. and Rehr, H. (1967). "Aging Ward Patients and the Hospital Social Work Department." *Journal of the American Geriatrics Society,* 15 (12).

Berkman, B. and Rehr, H. (1972). "Social Needs of the Hospitalized Elder: A Classification." *Social Work,* 17 (4), July.

Berkman, B., Rehr, H., and Rosenberg, G. (1980). "A Social Work Department Develops and Tests a Screening Mechanism to Identify High Social Risk Situations." *Social Work in Health Care,* 19 (11).

Berkman, B. and Weissman, A. (1983). "Applied Social Work Research." In *Social Work Issues in Health Care,* R. S. Miller and H. Rehr (eds.). New York: Prentice Hall, pp. 221-251.

Blumenfield, S. and Epstein, I. (2002). "Introduction: Promoting and Maintaining a Reflective Professional Staff in a Hospital-Based Social Work Department." In *Clinical Data-Mining in Practice-Based Research,* I. Epstein and S. Blumenfield (eds.). Binghamton, NY: The Haworth Press, p. 26.

Chernesky, R. and Lurie, A. (1976). "Developing a Quality Assurance Program." *Social Work in Health Care,* 1 (1).

Dana, B. (1983). "The Collaborative Process." In *Social Work Issues in Health Care,* R. Miller and H. Rehr (eds.). Englewood Cliffs, NJ: Prentice Hall.

Donabedian, A. (1973). *Aspects of Medical Care Administration.* Cambridge, MA: Harvard University Press.

End Stage Renal Disease Program Guidelines. (1977). Health Standards and Quality Bureau, Department of Health Education and Welfare, p. 1.

Epstein, I. (2001). "Using Available Clinical Information in Practice-Based Research: Mining for Silver While Dreaming of Gold." In *Clinical Data-Mining in Practice-Based Research,* I. Epstein and S. Blumenfield (eds.). Binghamton, NY: The Haworth Press, p. 96.

Feldman, R. (1992). "Foreword." In *Research Utilization in the New Social Services,* A. J. Grarse and I. Epstein (eds.). Binghamton NY: The Haworth Press.

Flexner, A. (1915). "Is Social Work a Profession?" National Conference of Charities and Corrections (Proceedings, 42nd Annual Meeting). Baltimore, MD, May 12-19.

Greene, R. (1976). *Assessing Quality in Medical Care.* Cambridge, MA: Ballinger Publication Co.

Jarrett, M. C. (1946). "A Method for Determining the Number of Social Workers Needed for Casework in a General Hospital." Social Service Division, Bellevue Hospital, New York.

Jenkins, S. (1990) "The Center Care Concept." *Practice and Research Newsletter,* CUSSW-JBFCS, Winter.

Johns Hopkins Department of Social Work (1992). Recording and Reporting Manual.

Kilbourne, E. (1988). "The Emergence of the Physician-Based Scientist." *Daedalus,* 15 (2), Spring.

Kirk, S. (1999). "Good Intentions Are Not Enough: Practice Guidelines for Social Work." *Research in Social Work Practice,* 9 (3).

Maluccio, A. N. (1979). *Learning from Clients.* New York: Free Press.

Maluccio, A. N. and Marlow, W. (1974). "The Case for the Contract." *Social Work,* 19 (1).

Morrison, B. J., Rehr, H., Rosenberg, G., and Davis, S. (1982). "Consumer Opinion Surveys: A Hospital Quality Assurance Measurement." *Quality Review Bulletin, 12*(2), pp. 13-17.

O'Neill, J. V. (2001). "Moving Research Findings in the Real World: Social Interventions in Health Care Research." *NASW News,* May.

Overton, A. (1960). "Taking Help from Our Clients." *Social Work,* 5 (2), April.

Perlman, R. (1975). *Consumers and Social Service.* New York: John Wiley.

PSRO Program Manual (1974). USDHEW, Office of Professional Standards Review. U.S. Government Printing Office, March 15.

Reardon, G. T., Blumenfeld, S., Weissman, A., and Rosenberg, G. (1988). "Findings and Implications from Pre-Admission Screening of Elderly Patients Waiting for Elective Surgery." *Social Work in Health Care,* 13 (3).

Rehr, H. (1979). "Looking to the Future." In *Professional Accountability for Social Work Practice,* H. Rehr (ed.). New York: Prodist, pp. 150-168.

Rehr, H. (1982). "Social Work Review Approaches to Evaluation and Analysis of Patient Care." *Quality Review Bulletin, 12*(2) Special Edition.

Rehr, H. (1989). "Using Clinical Satisfaction in an Indication of Effectiveness." In *Making Our Case,* B. Vourlekis and C. Leukefield (eds.). Silver Spring: NASW.

Rehr, H. (2001). "Foreword." In *Clinical Data-Mining,* I. Epstein and S. Blumenfield (eds.). Binghamton, NY: The Haworth Press.

Rehr, H., Rashbaum, W., Paneth, J., and Greenberg, M. (1962). "A Study of Extra-Marital Pregnancies." Monograph, The Mount Sinai Medical Center.

Rehr, H., Rashbaum, W., Paneth, J., and Greenberg, M. (1963). "Use of Social Services by Unmarried Mothers." *Children,* 10 (1), pp. 11-16.

Rehr, H., Rosenberg, G., and Blumenfield, S. (eds.) (1998). *Creative Social Work in Health Care.* New York: Springer Publishing Co.

Reid, W. (1980). "Research Strategies for Improving Individualized Services." In *Future of Social Work Research,* D. Fanshel (ed.). Washington, DC: NASW.

Reid, W. J. and Epstein, I. (1972). *Task-Centered Casework*. New York: Columbia University Press.

Schon, D. A. (1983). *The Reflective Practitioner*. New York: Basic Books.

Showers, N., Simon, E. P., Blumenfield, S., and Holden, G. (1995)."Predictions of Patient and Proxy Satisfaction with Discharge Planning." *Social Work in Health Care*, 22 (1).

Simon, E. P., Showers, N., Blumenfield, S., Holden, G., and Wu, X. (1995)."Delivery of Home Care Services After Discharge: What Really Happens." *Health and Social Work*, 20 (1), February.

Starfield, B. (1974). "Measurement of Outcome: A Proposed Scheme." *The Milbank Memorial Quarterly Health and Society*, 52 (1), Winter.

Sweet, A. and White E. (1961). "Social and Functional Rehabilitation of Patients with Severe Poliomyelitis." *Mount Sinai Journal of Medicine*, 28 (4).

Ware, I., Davis-Avery, A., and Stewart, A. (1978). "The Measurement and Meaning of Patient Satisfaction." *Health and Medical Care Services Review*, 1 (1).

Williams, T. F. (1988). "1987 Donald P. Kent Memorial Lecture." *The Gerontologist*, 28 (5).

Young, L. (1950). *Out-of-Wedlock*. New York: McGraw-Hill.

Chapter 8

Austin, D. (2000). "Greeting the Second Century: A Forward Look from a Historical Perspective." In *Social Work at the Millennium* (pp. 18-41), J. G. Hopps and R. Morris (eds.). New York: Free Press.

Bosch, S. J. and Deuschle, R. W. (1989). "Social Work: An Important Component of Community Medicine at Mount Sinai School of Medicine." *The Mount Sinai Journal of Medicine*, 56 (6), pp. 459-467.

Caroff, P. and Rehr, H. (1985). *A New Model in an Academic Practice Partnership*. Lexington, MA: Ginn Press.

Dana, B. (1983). "The Social Work–Community Medicine Connection." *Social Work in Health Care*, 8 (3), pp. 11-23.

Deuschle, K. W. (1970). "Community Medicine, 1970: Where the Action Is." *The Mount Sinai Medical Center News*, May-June, pp. 5-8.

End Stage Renal Disease Program (1953). Program Guidelines. Health Standards and Quality Bureau. Department of Education and Welfare.

McDermott, W. (1969). Keynote Address at Investure of Dr. Kurt W. Deuschle, as first Laurenburg Professor of Community Medicine, February 14. Unpublished.

Niss, B. and Aufses A. H. (2005). *Teaching Tomorrow's Medicine Today*. New York: New York University Press.

Niss, B. and Kase, N. G. (1989). "An Overview of the History of Mount Sinai School of Medicine and City University." *Mount Sinai*, June.

Peake, K., Brenner, B., and Rosenberg, G. (1998). "Community Development and Lay Participation." In *Creative Social Work in Health Care* (pp. 103-115).

H. Rehr, G. Rosenberg, and S. Blumenfeld (eds.). New York: Springer Publishing Co.

Rehr, H. and Rosenberg, G. (1984). "Today's Education for Today's Health Care Social Worker." In *Social Work Administration in Health Care,* A. Lurie and G. Rosenberg (eds.). Binghamton, NY: The Haworth Press, pp. 99-109.

Rehr, H. and Rosenberg, G. (2000). "Social Work and Health Care Today and Tomorrow." In *Social Work at the Millennium,* J. G. Hopps and R. Morris (eds.). New York: Free Press.

Rehr, H., Rosenberg, G., Walther, G. V., Showers, N., and Young, A. (1998). "Educating for Social-Health Care: Social Work Practitioners, Students and Other Health Care Professionals." In *Creative Social Work in Health Care* (pp. 129-157), H. Rehr, G. Rosenberg, and S. Blumenfeld (eds.). New York: Springer Publishing Co.

Siegel, D. (1969). Response to her investiture in the Edith J. Baerwald Professor in Community Medicine (Social Work). Unpublished.

Chapter 9

Berger, C. S. (1993). *Restructuring and Resizing: Strategies for Social Workers and Other Human Service Administrators in Health Care.* Chicago: American Hospital Association.

Indyk, D. and Bellville, R. (1995). "Linking Frontline Work and State-of-the-Art Knowledge: A Community Exchange System." *Journal of Care Management,* 4 (2), pp. 49-53.

McKay, M., Chasse, K. T., Palkoff, R., and McKinney, L. D. (2004). "Family-Level Impact of the CHAMP Family Program: A Community Collaborative Effort to Support Urban Families and Reduce Youth HIV Risk Exposure." *Family Process,* 43(1), pp. 77-91.

Midgley, J. (1990). "International Social Work: Learning from the Third World." *Social Work,* 35 (4), July, pp. 295-301.

Park, C. J. (2002). Editorial. *American Journal of Public Health,* 92(10), October, pp. 1582-1589.

Rehr, H., Rosenberg, G., and Blumenfield, S. (1993). "Enhancing Leadership Skills Through an International Exchange: The Mount Sinai Experience." *Social Work in Health Care,* 18 (3/4), pp. 13-33.

Chapter 10

Ancona-Berk, V. A. and Chalmers, T. C. (1996). "An Analysis of the Costs of Ambulatory and Inpatient Care." *American Journal of Public Health,* 76 (9), September.

Berger, C. S., Robbins, C., Lewis, M., Mizrahi, T., and Flex, S. (2003). "The Impact of Organizational Changes on Social Work Staffing in a Hospital Setting." *Social Work in Health Care*, 37 (1).

Berkman, B., Rehr, H., and Rosenberg, G. (1980). "A Social Work Department Develops and Tests a Screening Mechanism to Identify High Social Risk Situations." *Social Work in Health Care*, 19 (1).

Bloom, P. (2001). "Comments on Anti-Aging Research." Presentation at NYAM Conference, New York City, April.

Davis, K. (2004). Commonwealth Report, New York City, June 22.

Garfield, S. R. (1970). "The Delivery of Medical Care." *Scientific American*, 222 (4), April, pp. 15-23.

Kotelchuk, R. (1992). "New York City Health System: A Paradigm Under Siege." Presentation, The Mount Sinai Medical Center, April 2.

Mellor, J., with Rehr, H. and Social Work Section (2005). *Can My Eighties Be Like My Fifties*. New York: Springer Publishing Co.

Peake, K., Brenner, B., and Rosenberg, G. (1998). "Community Development and Lay Participation." In *Creative Social Work in Health Care* (Chapter 8), H. Rehr, G. Rosenberg, and S. Blumenfield (eds.). New York: Springer Publishing Co.

Pecukonis, E. V., Cornelius, L., and Parrish, M. (2003). "The Future of Health Social Work." *Social Work in Health Care*, 37 (3), pp. 1-15.

Rank, M. G. and Hutchison, W. S. (2000). "Analysis of Leadership in the Social Work Profession." *The Journal of Social Work Education*, 36, pp. 487-500.

Rehr, H. and Rosenberg, G. (1986). "Access to Social-Health Care: Implications for Social Work." In *Access to Social-Health Care*, H. Rehr (ed.). Lexington, MA: Ginn Press.

Rehr, H. and Rosenberg, G. (1991). "Social-Health Care: Problems and Predictions." In *The Changing Context of Social-Health Care* (pp. 97-120), H. Rehr and G. Rosenberg (eds.). Binghamton, NY: The Haworth Press.

Rehr, H., Rosenberg, G., and Blumenfield, S. (eds.) (1998). *Creative Social Work in Health Care: Clients, the Community and Your Organization*. New York: Springer Publishing Co.

Rehr, H., Rosenberg, G., and Blumenfield, S. (2000). "Social Work in Health Care Yesterday, Today and Tomorrow." In *Social Work at the Millennium* (pp. 24-25), S. J. G. Hopps and R. Morris (eds.). New York: Free Press.

Rosenberg, G. and Clarke, S. (eds.) (1987). "Social Work in Health Care Management: The Move to Leadership." Special Issue, *Social Work in Health Care*, 12 (3).

Rosenberg, G. and Katz, A. (2004). "Characteristics of Effective Leadership for Clinical Health Care Social Work Practice." In *Leadership in Health Care Social Work: Principles and Practice* (pp. 9-28), W. J. Spitzer (ed.). Richmond, VA: The Dietz Press.

Showers, N., Simon, E. P., Blumenfield, S., and Holden, G. (1995). "Predictions of Patient and Proxy Satisfaction with Discharge Plans." *Social Work in Health Care*, 22 (6).

Simon, E., Showers, N., Blumenfield, S., Holden, G., and Wu, X. (1995). "Delivery of Home Care Services After Discharge." *Health and Social Work,* 20 (1).

Thomas, L. (1977). "On the Science and Technology of Medicine." *Daedalus,* Winter.

Volland, P. (2001). "Social Work Education for Practice." Report, New York Academy of Medicine.

Index

Page numbers followed by the letter "f" indicate figures.

Abbott, Edith, 23, 108
Achilles' theragon, 13
"A Comprehensive Approach to Social Service in a Health Agency: A 1955 Perspective" (Siegel), 69-83
   balancing functions, 76-78
   blocks to balance, 78-80
   criteria for balance, 80-81
   functions and processes, 74-76
   past history, 70-72
   present pattern, 72-73
   references, 82
   work setting, 73-74
Addams, Jane, 23, 90
After-Care Movement in Psychiatry, 22-23
AIDS, 30, 148
ALCS. *See* Arthur Lehman Counseling Services (ALCS)
American Association of Hospital Social Workers, 25
American Medical Association, 21, 26
American medicine
   and emergence of social work profession, 17-32
      fiscal factors, 29-31
      forerunners of medical social work, 20
      introduction, 17-19
      medical innovations, 27-28
      physician specialization, 31
      social work connects to medicine, 20-32
American Red Cross, 24

"An Aspiring Researcher Begins at Mount Sinai" (Berkman), 97-99
"An Experiment in Staff Education Conducted at the Social Service Department of the Mount Sinai Hospital: A 1932 Perspective" (Mendelsohn), 64-69
Aron, Jack, 58
Aron, Jane, 58
Arthur Lehman Counseling Service (ALCS), 59
Aufses, A. H., 125
Auslander, Gail, 106

Baehr, George, 49, 54, 56, 64
Baker Memorial Hospital Training Centers, 25
Balance, 76-82
   achieving, 76-78
   blocks to, 78-80
   criteria for, 80-81
   issues, 81-82
Bellevue Hospital, 19, 35, 48
Berkman, Barbara, 92, 97-99
Berkman-Rehr Problem Classification, 94
Blackwell, Elizabeth, 20, 36
Blizzard, Sir William, 14
Blue Cross, 27
Blumenfield, Susan, 55, 59, 106
Brookdale Center for Continuing Education, 56, 121

Cabot, Richard, 22, 36, 115
Cannon, I. M., 24-25
Cannon, Ida, 115
Caregivers and Professional Partnership (CAPP), 41
Center for Multicultural and Community Affairs, 41
Charity Organization Society, 13
Chasse, K. T., 139
Child Guidance Clinic, 23
Children's Health Clinic, 48
Christians, early medicine, 10-11
Clarke, Sylvia, 60
Client satisfaction, 94-95
Clinical data-mining, 105-106
Cole, Rebecca, 36
Columbia University, 19
Communicard, 41
Community medicine
    and social work connection, 113-125
        background, 114-117
        community practice, 121-123
        conclusion, 124-125
        division of social work, 117-118
        research, 123-124
        role in medical education, 118-120
        schools of social work, 120-121
Compliance, 25
Comprehensive Breast Service, 40
Continuous quality improvement (CQI), 89-91, 92, 94
Cook, Mrs. Alfred J., 54
Cornelius, L., 159
Cornell Medical College, 19, 35
CQI. *See* continuous quality improvement (CQI)
Crusaders, early medicine, 11
Cuzzi, Lawrence, 99-101

Daniel, Anne, 20
de Paul, Vincent, 13-14
Deregulation, of health care, 29-30
Deuschle, Kurt W., 113-114
Diagnosis-related groups (DRGs), 88, 145-146

Dix, Dorothea, 23
Donabedian, A., 111
Donabedian, Avedis, 88
DRGs. *See* Diagnosis-related groups (DRGs)

EAP. *See* Employee Assistance Program (EAP)
Edith J. Baerwald Professor of Community Medicine (Social Work), 58, 115, 116
Edith K. Ehrman Health Education Center, 60
Elizabethan Poor Law of 1598, 12
ELP. *See* Enhanced Leadership Program (ELP)
Emerson, Charles, 22
Employee Assistance Program (EAP), 40, 60
Enhanced Leadership Program (ELP), 130-138
    creation, 130-131
    curriculum, 134-135
    exchange program, 133, 136-138
    fiscal crisis and, 131-132
    gains as result of, 137-138
    key concerns of social work leaders, 132-134
    limitation, 138
    means, 131
    objectives, 131, 135-136
Epstein, Irwin, 59, 94, 101-107

Family Resource Center Library, 40-41
Fizdale, Ruth, 59
Flexner, Abraham, 19, 24, 35, 85, 87
Friendly visitor, 22, 23
"From Evaluation Methodologist to Clinical Data-Miner: Finding Treasure Through Practice-Based Research" (Epstein), 101-107

Gantt, Ami, 104
Garfield, S. R., 158
General Motors, 26-27
"Going Across Town and Out into the World" (Holden), 107-111
Goldwater, S. S., 48
Gopher Resources for Social Workers, 109
Greeks
 early medicine, 9-10
 life force, 9
 psyche, 9
Green Box, 39
Greenthal, Jennie, 48

Harvard Medical School, 19, 35
Health and Social Work (journal), 60-61
Health Careers Pipeline Mentoring Program, 41
Health Professions Education Act, 27
Hebrews
 early medicine, 8-9
 public health, 9
Hill-Burton Act, 27
Hippocrates, 10
Hobby, Oveta Culp, 44
Holden, Gary, 107-111
Holocaust Survivors Project, 41
Hoover, Herbert, 24
Hopkins, John, 19
Hospital almoner, 14, 22
Hospital Corps and Visitors Guide, 41
Hospitals
 fiscal crisis of late-twentieth century, 29
 history, 9, 10, 11
Hunter College School of Social Work–Mount Sinai Consortium, 42, 56
Hutchison, W. S., 159

Information for Practice (IP), 109
International Conference of Social Work in Health and Mental Health, 56
International Educational Institute in Social-Health, 140-141
International Enhancement of Social Work Leadership Program at Mount Sinai, 56
IP. *See Information for Practice* (IP)

James, George, 113
Janover, Betty, 54
Jarrett, Mary, 92
Jenkins, S., 97
Jews' Hospital, 33-35, 114. *See also* Mount Sinai Hospital
Johnson, Rose, 48
Joint Commission of Accreditation of Health Organizations (JCAHO), 59, 88, 89
Joubert, Lynette, 106
Journal of Social Work and Mental Health, 61
Juvenile Diabetes Teaching Service, 41

Kaiser Permanete Program, 157-158

Leadership Enhancement and Exchange Program, 106
Lehman, Mrs. Herbert, 39
Leplin, Pauline, 54
Levinson, Anna, 54
Lewis, Myrna, 107
Loch, Charles, 14
Lokshin, Helen, 99-100
London Charity Organization Society, 14
Luce, Claire Booth, 44
Lyons, Albert, 5

Maemonides, 11
Maluccio, A. N., 94
Marine Hospital Service, 18

Markowitz, Matilda, 54
Marlow, W., 94
Massachusetts General Hospital, 19, 22, 35, 48
Maternal and Child Health Service, 26
McDermott, W., 121-122
McKay, M., 139
McKinney, L. D., 139
Medicaid, 21, 26, 148
Medicare, 21, 26, 148
Medicine
   American. *See* American medicine
   community. *See* Community medicine
Medicine: An Illustrated History (Lyons and Petrucelli), 5
Mendelsohn, Fannie, née Lissauer, 50, 52, 53, 61, 63, 64-69
Methadone Maintenance, 41
Meyer, Adolph, 22, 23
Midgeley, J., 139
Mom and Tots Program, 41
Moss, Celia, 53
Mount Sinai Auxiliary Board, 34, 37-42
   Caregivers and Professional Partnership, 41
   creation of social services department, 39
   education of health care providers, 42
   formation of, 37-38
   funding, 39
   gift shop, 39
   innovative projects, 39-40
   patient care projects, 40-41
   public health policy issues, 41
   response to local and national social conditions, 40
   roles assumed by, 38-39
   women and, 42-45
Mount Sinai Hospital. *See also* Jews' Hospital
   social work service department, 47-62
      1927 annual report, 50-52
      1952 department review, 52-53

Mount Sinai Hospital, social work service department *(continued)*
      accountability, 59
      changing face of health care, 61-62
      Children's Health Clinic, 48
      collaboration with medical interns, 48-49
      expansion of work, 50
      as field unit for social work students, 58
      fiscal difficulties, 61
      growth, 47
      initial services offered, 48
      manual for staff orientation, 52
      marketing of social services, 59-60
      publications, 60-61
      range of current services, 55-58
      staff education, 52
      women activists who initiated, 47
   use of European type of scientific medicine, 35
   women who socialized the institution, 33-45
      medical model of care, 35
      Mount Sinai Auxiliary Board, 34, 37-42
      summary, 42-45
Mount Sinai Medical School, 58
Murray M. Rosenberg Applied Social Work Research Center, 56

National Academies of Science and of Practice, 111
National Health Insurance Act, 14
National Institute of Mental Health (NIMH), 103
National Institutes of Health, 27, 111
New York Hospital, 19, 35
New York Infirmary for Women and Children, 20, 36
Nightingale, Florence, 12-13, 87
NIMH. *See* National Institute of Mental Health (NIMH)

Niss, B., 125
Nursing, 12-13

Osler, William, 22

Pain Management Program, 41
Palkoff, R., 139
Palliative Care Project, 41
Parrish, M., 159
Patient Representative Program, 40, 122
Patroclus, 13
Peabody, Francis, 22
Pecukonis, E. V., 159
Pennsylvania's Hospital and University, 19, 35
Pet-Assisted Therapy Program, 41
Petrucelli, R. J., 5
Physical Medicine, 27
Popper, Hans, 113
Practice-based studies, 90-97
Pratt, Joseph, 22
Professional review committees (PROs), 88
Provident Dispensaries, 14
Psychoanalytic theory, and social work, 26
Public health
  Hebrew form, 9
  in seventeenth century, 12
Public Health Service, 27
Putnam, William, 22

Rank, M. G., 159
RBRVS. *See* Resource-Based Relative Value Scales (RBRVS)
REAP. *See* Resource Entitlement and Advocacy Program (REAP)
Regensberg, Jeanette, 42
Rehr, Helen, 55, 59, 92, 97, 99, 160
Reid, W. J., 94

Resource-Based Relative Value Scales (RBRVS), 146
Resource Entitlement and Advocacy Program (REAP), 40, 122
Reynolds, Bertha, 90
Richmond, Mary, 24, 90
Right to health care, 2, 3, 30, 143
Romans, early medicine, 10
Roosevelt, Eleanor, 44
Roosevelt, Franklin D., 26
Rosenberg, Gary, 55, 59-60, 98, 99, 102-104, 107, 160
Rosner, D. K., 19, 35
Rusk, Howard, 27

Safety net concept, 30
Sanitary visitor, 36
Secondary Education Through Health Program (SETH), 40
Siegel, Doris, 53-54, 61, 62, 63-64, 69-83, 122
Social Darwinism, 34
Social Diagnosis (Richmond), 24
Social-health program, proposed, 158f
Social reform movement, 23-24
Social Security, 26
Social service hostel, 33
Social work
  American medicine and emergence of profession, 17-32
    fiscal factors, 29-31
    forerunners of medical social work, 20
    introduction, 17-19
    medical innovations, 27-28
    physician specialization, 31
    social work connects to medicine, 20-32
  community medicine and, 113-125
    background, 114-117
    community practice, 121-123
    conclusion, 124-125
    division of social work, 117-118
    research, 123-124

Social work, community medicine and *(continued)*
    role in medical education, 118-120
    schools of social work, 120-121
  early medicine and, 7-15
    as ancient history, 7
    Arabs, 11
    beginning of medical social services, 13-14
    beginning of modern medicine, 14-15
    Christians, 10-11
    Crusaders, 11
    Greeks, 9-10
    healers, 7-8
    Hebrews, 8-9
    hospital almoner, 14
    hospitals, 9
    Middle Ages, 11
    public health, 12
    regulation of medical practice, 8
    relief organizations, 13
    Romans, 10
    social development breakdown, 15
    supernatural causation, 7
    therapy, 13
    women as healers, 12-13
  functions, 155f
  globalization, 127-142
    developing countries' needs, 138-140
    Enhanced Leadership Program, 130-138
    international exchange among social work leaders, 127-129
    other enhancement of leadership programs, 141-142
    Western social workers' needs, 140-141
  health care challenges, 1-6
    economics, 1-2
    excess and deprivation, 2
    history of medicine and social work, 4-6
    key concerns, 4

Social work, health care challenges *(continued)*
    shift in health care focus, 4
    social-health gains, 3-4
    societal problems, 2-3
  past shaping present practice, 63-83
    introduction, 63-64
    Mendelsohn's presentation, 64-69
    Siegel's presentation, 69-83
  proposed social-health program, 158f
  research in health care, 85-112
    "An Aspiring Researcher Begins at Mount Sinai" (Berkman), 97-99
    background, 87-90
    conclusion, 111-112
    "From Evaluation Methodologist to Clinical Data-Miner: Finding Treasure Through Practice-Based Research" (Epstein), 101-107
    "Going Across Town and Out into the World" (Holden), 107-111
    objectives, 85-86
    practice-based studies, 90-97
    premise, 86-87
    "Thirty-Five Years of Social Work at Elmhurst Hospital" (Cuzzi), 99-101
  social-health challenge, 143-163
    conclusions, 160-163
    economics of health care delivery, 144-146
    future, 155-160
    new millennium, 147-150
    social policy, 150-154
"Social Work and Health Care Yesterday, Today and Tomorrow" (Rehr and Rosenberg), 160-163
Social Work in Health Care (journal), 60-61
Spiegel, Frances, 54
Spielberg, Steven, 108

Spinal Cord Project, 40
Starbright Foundation, 108
State Charities Aid Association, 44

The Second Sex (De Beauvoir), 44
"Thirty-Five Years of Social Work at Elmhurst Hospital" (Cuzzi), 99-101
Thomas, Lewis, 13
Translational research, 109
Tripodi, Tony, 102
Tuberculosis, 33

Uniform Hospital Discharge Data System (UHDDS), 89
University of New York Medical School, 19, 35

War on Poverty, 21, 30
Weissman, Andrew, 60, 61
White House Conference for Child Health and Protection, 24, 25
Williams, T. Franklin, 95
Women
    acceptance into medical profession, 36-37
    as healers in early medicine, 12-13
    Mount Sinai Auxiliary Board and, 42-45
    roles in serving the sick poor, 36
    traditional values in nineteenth century, 36-37
World Wide Web Resources for Social Workers (WWWRSW), 109

Zakrewski, Marie, 20

Order a copy of this book with this form or online at:
http://www.haworthpress.com/store/product.asp?sku=5717

THE SOCIAL WORK–MEDICINE RELATIONSHIP
100 Years at Mount Sinai

_____ in hardbound at $39.95 (ISBN-13: 978-0-7890-3076-4; ISBN-10: 0-7890-3076-4)

_____ in softbound at $24.95 (ISBN-13: 978-0-7890-3077-1; ISBN-10: 0-7890-3077-2)

Or order online and use special offer code HEC25 in the shopping cart.

COST OF BOOKS_____

☐ **BILL ME LATER:** (Bill-me option is good on US/Canada/Mexico orders only; not good to jobbers, wholesalers, or subscription agencies.)

☐ Check here if billing address is different from shipping address and attach purchase order and billing address information.

POSTAGE & HANDLING_____
(US: $4.00 for first book & $1.50 for each additional book)
(Outside US: $5.00 for first book & $2.00 for each additional book)

Signature_____

SUBTOTAL_____

☐ **PAYMENT ENCLOSED:** $_____

IN CANADA: ADD 7% GST_____

☐ **PLEASE CHARGE TO MY CREDIT CARD.**

STATE TAX_____
(NJ, NY, OH, MN, CA, IL, IN, PA, & SD residents, *add appropriate local sales tax*)

☐ Visa ☐ MasterCard ☐ AmEx ☐ Discover
☐ Diner's Club ☐ Eurocard ☐ JCB

Account #_____

FINAL TOTAL_____
(If paying in Canadian funds, convert using the current exchange rate, UNESCO coupons welcome)

Exp. Date_____

Signature_____

Prices in US dollars and subject to change without notice.

NAME_____
INSTITUTION_____
ADDRESS_____
CITY_____
STATE/ZIP_____
COUNTRY_____ COUNTY (NY residents only)_____
TEL_____ FAX_____
E-MAIL_____

May we use your e-mail address for confirmations and other types of information? ☐ Yes ☐ No
We appreciate receiving your e-mail address and fax number. Haworth would like to e-mail or fax special discount offers to you, as a preferred customer. **We will never share, rent, or exchange your e-mail address or fax number.** We regard such actions as an invasion of your privacy.

Order From Your Local Bookstore or Directly From
The Haworth Press, Inc.
10 Alice Street, Binghamton, New York 13904-1580 • USA
TELEPHONE: 1-800-HAWORTH (1-800-429-6784) / Outside US/Canada: (607) 722-5857
FAX: 1-800-895-0582 / Outside US/Canada: (607) 771-0012
E-mail to: orders@haworthpress.com

For orders outside US and Canada, you may wish to order through your local sales representative, distributor, or bookseller.
For information, see http://haworthpress.com/distributors

(Discounts are available for individual orders in US and Canada only, not booksellers/distributors.)

PLEASE PHOTOCOPY THIS FORM FOR YOUR PERSONAL USE.
http://www.HaworthPress.com